THE **JUICE AND ZEST** BOOK

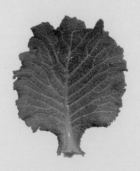

THE
JUICE AND ZEST
BOOK

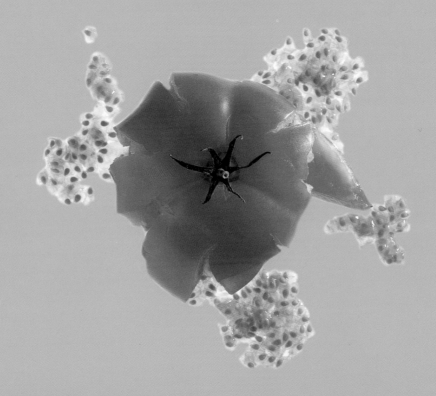

RECIPES FOR HEALING & VITALITY

ANNA SELBY

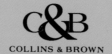

COLLINS & BROWN

First published in Great Britain in 2000
by Collins & Brown Limited
London House
Great Eastern Wharf
Parkgate Road
London SW11 4NQ

Distributed in the United States and Canada by Sterling Publishing Co,
387 Park Avenue South, New York, NY 10016, USA

1 3 5 7 9 8 6 4 2

British Library Cataloguing-in-Publication Data:
A catalogue record for this book
is available from the British Library.

ISBN 1 85585 786 3

Editor: Amy Corzine
Designer: Sue Miller
Jacket design: Alison Lee
Photography: Sian Irvine

Reproduction by Classic Scan, Singapore
Printed and bound in Hong Kong by Toppan

SAFETY NOTE: This book is written for those interested in nutrition and its
effects on health and lifestyle. Every effort has been made to ensure that the
contents are accurate and current, but medical and nutritional knowledge are
constantly advancing and this book is not intended to replace expert medical
advice and diagnosis. The author and publisher cannot be held liable for any
errors or omissions in the book, or for any actions that may be taken as a
consequence of using it.

Contents

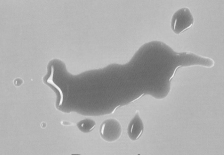

Part 1

Juice Facts 6
Why juice? **8**
Introducing juices into your day **20**
How to juice **32**

Part 2

Juice Recipes 42
100 recipes **44**

Part 3

Health Directory 82
Juices for ailments **84**

Part 4

Juice Plans 98
Juice fasting **100**
The one-day plan **102**
The three-day plan **110**

Useful addresses **124**
Further reading and
acknowledgements **125**
Index **126**

juice

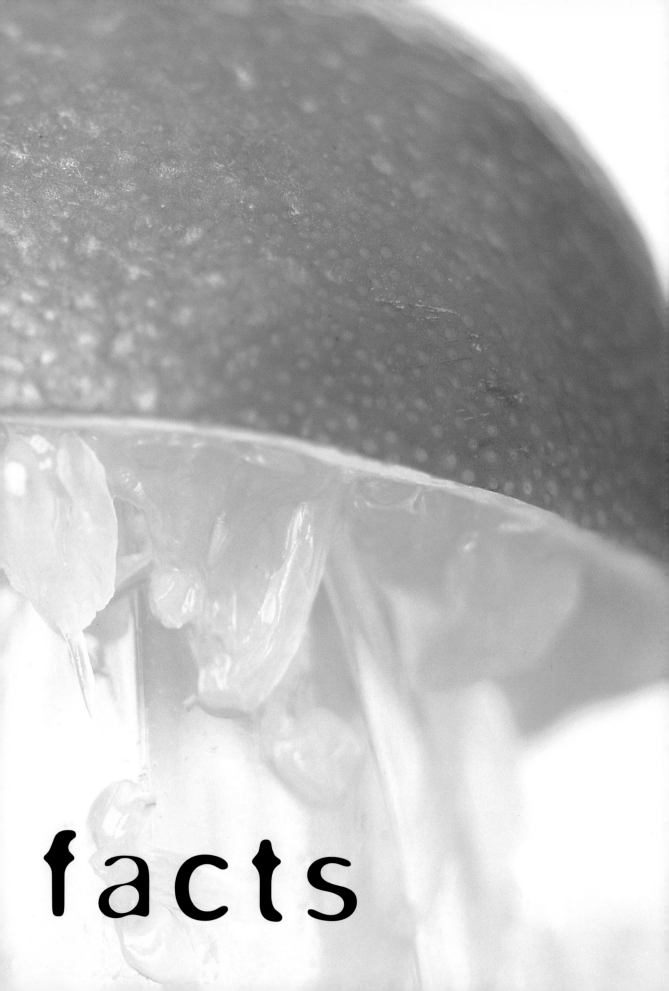

facts

The

inevitable question you are

asked when you tell someone that you

regularly drink fruit and vegetable juices is:

"Why don't you just eat the fruit and vegetables?"

There are quite a few answers to this. One is that, as

everyone knows, fruits and vegetables are packed with vital

nutrients in the form of vitamins, minerals and enzymes. These

Why juice?

are all necessary for good health. The British government's

recommendation that everyone should have five portions of fruit or

vegetables every day is well-advertized, but too rarely followed. So the

first and simplest answer to this question is that it is a lot easier to

drink a glass of carrot juice than to munch your way through a pound

of carrots! Another is that the body absorbs juice a great deal more

rapidly and efficiently than it does food, or mineral and vitamin

supplements. Yet another is that juices are, by definition, raw,

and so none of their vital nutrients are destroyed by the

cooking process. Juices are cleansing, healing,

energizing and rejuvenating, but perhaps the

best reason of all for drinking them is

that they are, quite simply,

delicious.

Juicing for
optimum health

Many people think of their bodies in the way they think of their cars. Give them enough fuel and the occasional service, and they shouldn't break down too often – and if a breakdown does occur, it's off to the mechanic for a quick fix.

Of course, our bodies are not machines, but living, growing organisms that are continually renewing and repairing themselves on a cellular level. In order to function at optimum level, they require the best possible nutrition.

Unfortunately, most of the time this simply doesn't happen. This is partly due to the pace of modern life. When we must travel long distances to jobs, and then work increasingly longer hours after we get there, run our homes, bring up our children, and find time to see our friends and families, something just has to go. And one of the first is spending hours in the kitchen preparing healthy meals, however good for us they may be. As a consequence, we eat more and more processed convenience foods from supermarkets and junk food from fast-food chains. These almost always have too much salt, fat and sugar in them, not to mention preservatives, colourings and flavourings, all of which are nutritionally worthless at best, and damaging at worst.

PROTECTING AGAINST DISEASE

Just how harmful the effects of poor nutrition can be has been acknowledged by the World Health Organization. It has found that around eighty-five per cent of adult cancers are avoidable and, of these, half are related to dietary deficiencies. Many of these cancers are found, not in those parts of the world that suffer great poverty and starvation, but in the rich, developed world where we eat, not too little, but too much. The problem is that the food we eat is nutritionally poor; the nutrients we need have been processed out of it.

One of the most important dietary findings of the World Health Organization is that there are particular nutrients that are vital for good health. These are the vitamins A (beta-carotene from vegetable sources), C and E, together with the mineral selenium. They are known as antioxidants, and their protective powers are widely recognized. This protection extends not only against minor infections but also more serious conditions, including cancer and heart disease. Antioxidants are believed by many to protect against premature ageing as well.

SUPER SCAVENGERS

Antioxidants destroy or disable free radicals – electrochemically unbalanced molecules – that our bodies generate. Free radicals are linked to a wide variety of sources, including pollution, stress, overeating, pesticides, cigarettes, certain foods, and drugs. Once generated, they react with other, previously healthy, molecules, making them unstable, too. Thus, a never-ending chain reaction is set up, leading to a process of cellular destruction and disease.

This process is halted when antioxidants destroy or transform free radicals. Providing our bodies with antioxidants is one of the best forms of preventative health care we can take.

How juices
fight disease

As mentioned already, antioxidants are at the forefront of the body's defence system. The main antioxidants are vitamins A, C and E, together with selenium, but many of the B-complex vitamins, as well as zinc, enzymes and certain amino acids also have antioxidant properties. It is, of course, simple enough to find any or all of these in the form of pills that can be taken on a regular basis, and these, indisputably, have a beneficial effect. However, one of the interesting findings that has emerged from research into antioxidants is that their protective effect increases when they are taken together rather than on their own. And, while you may think it wise to take a multivitamin and mineral supplement, an ideal nutritional balance occurs naturally in fruit and vegetables already.

ONGOING RESEARCH
It is worth noting that nutrition is a constantly developing science, and new findings are being brought to light all the time. After all, vitamin C itself was discovered only in the 1920s! So, while we have recently acquired all of this essential new information on antioxidants and how they work together, they may be only a part of the picture and there could well be other, more subtle, reasons why the whole and complex nature of the fresh nutrients in fruit and vegetables make them so beneficial to our health.

Fruit and vegetables are certainly among the best sources of antioxidants. However, antioxidants, along with many other nutrients, can easily be destroyed by cooking, so fruit and vegetables are most effective in a raw state. This is one of the reasons why juices are so beneficial. Because they are raw (including the juice of vegetables which you would probably never consider eating raw, such as turnips or beetroot), all of the nutrients are at their peak. Also, it is far easier to drink large quantities of carrot juice than to eat bunches of carrots throughout the day. Five average-sized raw carrots, for instance, will give you around 20,000 microgrammes of beta-carotene, which the body will transform into vitamin A. A glass of carrot juice will do the job equally well – without the jaw-ache!

HEALTH AND LONGEVITY
The only thing that is missing from juice is the fibre that is found in the whole fruit or vegetable from which the juice is made. For this reason, it is important to include whole raw foods in your diet. Don't think of juices as a substitute for them, but more of a vital addition. Even though juices contain no fibre, they have a powerful cleansing effect on the body and help to remove toxins from the digestive tract. As a means of boosting immune processes, detoxifying the system and guarding against disease and premature ageing, juices are hard to beat. For the simple reason that they are liquid, it is much easier for the body to absorb and assimilate them rapidly, even if you have a sluggish or problematic digestive system.

There may even be links between juices and our mental and emotional health. While this is

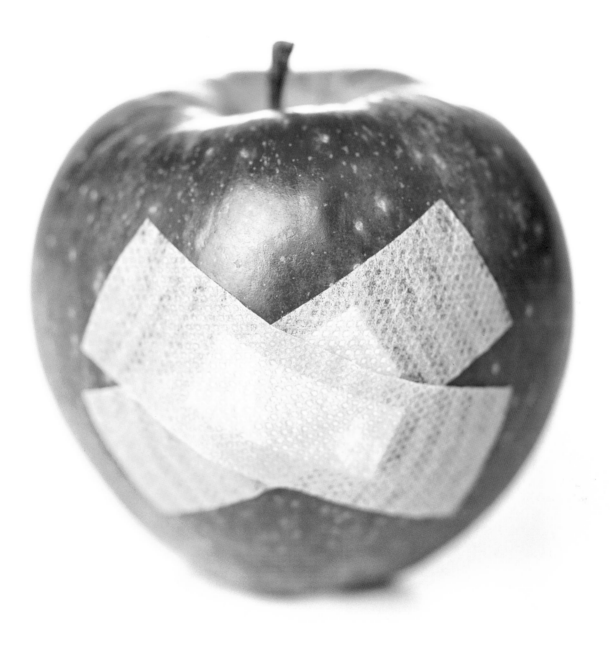

still an area that is undergoing research, it seems possible that many problems – from senility to schizophrenia to depression – may be linked to specific nutritional deficiencies of, for example, zinc, vitamin B1 and certain amino acids.

If further persuasion were needed, many long-term regular juicers believe that it also improves the look of their skin. Wrinkles and lines, so often the target of expensive moisturizers, soften to leave the skin looking smoother and younger. Juices are also thought to keep fingernails and bones strong and may actually make you live longer. Norman Walker, who pioneered juicing in the United States, is said by some to have lived to the age of 113!

A–Z of
vitamins and minerals

Vitamin	Benefit/function	Found in
A (beta-carotene)	One of the main antioxidants, vitamin A boosts the immune system, builds strong teeth, hair and bones and protects and strengthens the respiratory and digestive systems.	Found as vitamin A only in dairy foods, eggs, fish and liver, but the body converts beta-carotene into vitamin A. Beta-carotene can be found in carrots, dark green leafy vegetables, red and yellow peppers, pumpkins, sweet potatoes, oranges, melons, mangoes, apricots and peaches.
B1 (thiamine)	Vital for metabolizing starchy foods for energy, it benefits the muscles and nervous system.	Garlic, leeks, cauliflower, oranges, pineapples.
B2 (riboflavin)	Vital for metabolizing fats into energy, it benefits the skin, hair and nails.	Apricots, peaches, cherries, broccoli, spinach, watercress.
B3 (niacin)	Used in metabolizing various foods to produce energy, it strengthens the nervous and digestive systems.	Bean sprouts, parsley, red peppers, grapes, strawberries, passion fruit.
B5 (pantothenic acid)	Another vitamin used in metabolism to produce energy.	Watermelon, all berries, celery, broccoli, sweet potatoes.
B6 (pyridoxine)	Important for metabolizing protein and for the health of the skin, and the nervous and immune systems.	Bananas, watermelon, blackcurrants, leeks, sweet potatoes, green peppers.
B12	Vital for the metabolism of iron and a healthy nervous system and blood cells.	The body can make its own B12; otherwise, it is found in seaweed.
C	A powerful antioxidant, immune system booster, wound healer, protector against heart disease, cancer and other degenerative disorders. It aids the body in its absorption of iron – particularly necessary for those who smoke, are ill or are under stress.	Green leafy vegetables, citrus fruits, blackcurrants, mangoes, pawpaws, pineapples, parsley, peppers, tomatoes, potatoes.
D	Strengthens bones, and facilitates the absorption of calcium and phosphorus.	Made by the body from sunlight.
E	A powerful antioxidant, it protects cells and the circulation and immune systems, and prevents premature ageing.	All dark green leafy vegetables.
Folic acid	Essential for pregnant women, this protects against spina bifida in unborn babies and strengthens the nervous system and blood cells.	Beetroot, broccoli, cabbages, melons, citrus fruits.
K	Essential for blood clotting.	Green leafy vegetables.

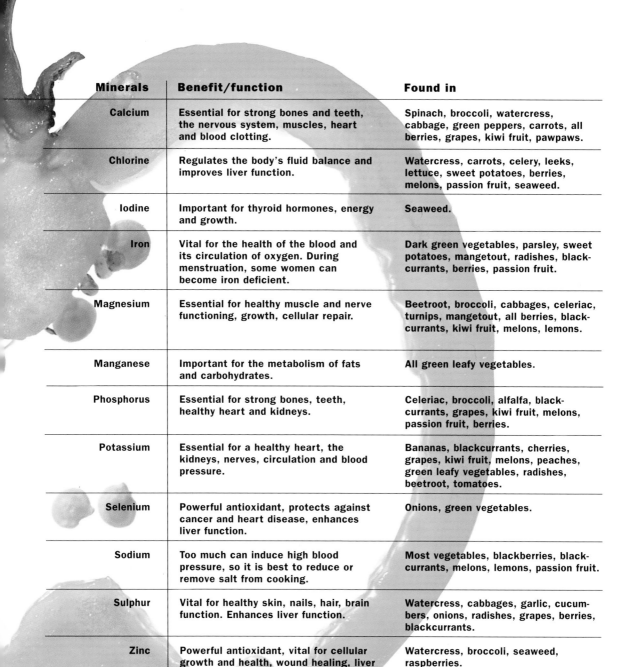

Minerals	Benefit/function	Found in
Calcium	Essential for strong bones and teeth, the nervous system, muscles, heart and blood clotting.	Spinach, broccoli, watercress, cabbage, green peppers, carrots, all berries, grapes, kiwi fruit, pawpaws.
Chlorine	Regulates the body's fluid balance and improves liver function.	Watercress, carrots, celery, leeks, lettuce, sweet potatoes, berries, melons, passion fruit, seaweed.
Iodine	Important for thyroid hormones, energy and growth.	Seaweed.
Iron	Vital for the health of the blood and its circulation of oxygen. During menstruation, some women can become iron deficient.	Dark green vegetables, parsley, sweet potatoes, mangetout, radishes, black-currants, berries, passion fruit.
Magnesium	Essential for healthy muscle and nerve functioning, growth, cellular repair.	Beetroot, broccoli, cabbages, celeriac, turnips, mangetout, all berries, black-currants, kiwi fruit, melons, lemons.
Manganese	Important for the metabolism of fats and carbohydrates.	All green leafy vegetables.
Phosphorus	Essential for strong bones, teeth, healthy heart and kidneys.	Celeriac, broccoli, alfalfa, black-currants, grapes, kiwi fruit, melons, passion fruit, berries.
Potassium	Essential for a healthy heart, the kidneys, nerves, circulation and blood pressure.	Bananas, blackcurrants, cherries, grapes, kiwi fruit, melons, peaches, green leafy vegetables, radishes, beetroot, tomatoes.
Selenium	Powerful antioxidant, protects against cancer and heart disease, enhances liver function.	Onions, green vegetables.
Sodium	Too much can induce high blood pressure, so it is best to reduce or remove salt from cooking.	Most vegetables, blackberries, black-currants, melons, lemons, passion fruit.
Sulphur	Vital for healthy skin, nails, hair, brain function. Enhances liver function.	Watercress, cabbages, garlic, cucumbers, onions, radishes, grapes, berries, blackcurrants.
Zinc	Powerful antioxidant, vital for cellular growth and health, wound healing, liver and hormone function.	Watercress, broccoli, seaweed, raspberries.

Top 20 fruits for juicing

Fruits	Rich in	Traces of	Benefits
Apple	Beta-carotene, folic acid, vitamin C, calcium, magnesium, phosphorus, potassium, pectin.	Copper, zinc and vitamins B1, B2, B3, B6 and E.	A delicious, sweet juice that mixes with just about everything. Antioxidant, cleansing (particularly for the digestive system) and boosts the immune system.
Blackberry	Beta-carotene, vitamins C and E, calcium, magnesium, phosphorus, potassium, sodium.	B vitamins, iron, copper.	Delicious, dark purple juice that mixes well. Powerful antioxidant, immune system booster.
Pear	Beta-carotene, folic acid, vitamin C, calcium, magnesium, phosphorus, potassium, pectin.	B vitamins, copper, iron, manganese, zinc.	A sweet, light juice that is very powerful as an antioxidant, immune system booster and detoxifier. Energizing, good intestinal cleanser, reduces cholesterol.
Blackcurrant	Beta-carotene, vitamins C and E, calcium, magnesium, phosphorus, potassium.	B vitamins, copper, iron.	Strong, sweet taste, best mixed with apple. Powerful antioxidant, anti-inflammatory, and immune system booster.
Apricot	Beta-carotene, folic acid, calcium, magnesium, iron, potassium, and vitamins C, B3 and B5.	Copper, and vitamins B1, B2 and B6.	Another deliciously sweet juice which needs to be mixed, as only a little juice comes from the fruit. Antioxidant, cleansing, boosts the immune system.
Pawpaw	Beta-carotene, vitamin C, papain, calcium, magnesium, phosphorus, potassium, flavonoids.	B vitamins, iron, zinc.	Delicious, thick juice that needs to be mixed well. Antioxidant, immune system booster, energizer, cleanses and soothes the digestive tract.
Grapes	Vitamins C and E, calcium, magnesium, phosphorus, potassium, flavonoids.	B vitamins, copper, iron, zinc.	Sweet, thick juice that is a powerful antioxidant immune system booster and detoxifier for the liver, kidneys and intestines, and is good for skin.
Cherry	Beta-carotene, vitamin C, folic acid, calcium, magnesium, phosphorus, potassium, flavonoids.	B vitamins, iron, zinc.	Deliciously sweet juice, but it does not yield much liquid and is time-consuming to prepare, so it is best diluted. Another powerful antioxidant and immune system booster.
Kiwi fruit	Beta-carotene, vitamin C, calcium, magnesium, phosphorus, potassium, bioflavonoids.	B vitamins, iron.	Light green juice, good for mixes. Very powerful antioxidant immune system booster, cleanser and energizer.
Mango	Beta-carotene, calcium, vitamin C, magnesium, potassium, flavonoids.	B vitamins, copper, iron, zinc.	Thick, sweet juice. Energizing antioxidant immune system booster. Breaks down proteins in the digestive system.

Fruits	Rich in	Traces of	Benefits
Melon	Beta-carotene, folic acid, vitamin C, calcium, chlorine, magnesium, phosphorus, potassium.	B vitamins, vitamin E, copper, iron, zinc.	Sweet, fragrant juice. Antioxidant, cleansing, diuretic.
Peach	Beta-carotene, folic acid, vitamins B3 and C, flavonoids, calcium, magnesium, phosphorus, potassium.	B vitamins, iron, zinc.	Delicious, sweet, thick juice. Antioxidant, immune system boosting, energizing.
Orange	Beta-carotene, folic acid, iron, calcium, potassium and vitamins B1, B6 and C.	B vitamins, vitamin E, zinc.	Delicious juice, whether alone or mixed. Powerful antioxidant, immune system booster and cleanser for the liver and kidneys.
Nectarine	Beta-carotene, vitamin C, folic acid, calcium, magnesium, phosphorus, potassium.	B vitamins, iron, zinc.	Sweet, thick, energizing antioxidant juice.
Watermelon	Beta-carotene, folic acid, vitamins B5 and C, calcium, magnesium, phosphorus, potassium.	B vitamins, iron, zinc.	The high water content of this very liquid juice tends to make it overflow the juicer! Antioxidant, detoxing, diuretic.
Banana	Beta-carotene, vitamin C, folic acid, magnesium, calcium, phosphorus, potassium.	Iron, B vitamins, zinc.	Although very little juice comes from a banana, its flavour and smell make it worth using in mixtures. It's very thick and needs to be stirred well or it will sink to the bottom. Great energy booster.
Pineapple	Beta-carotene, folic acid, vitamin C, bromelian, calcium, magnesium, phosphorus, potassium.	B vitamins, iron, zinc.	Delicious, fragrant, thick juice. Antioxidant immune system booster that improves protein digestion and cleanses and protects the intestines.
Plum	Beta-carotene, folic acid, vitamins C and E, calcium, magnesium, phosphorus, potassium.	B vitamins, iron.	Sweet, fragrant juice that is an antioxidant immune system booster, which stimulates the digestive process.
Raspberry	Beta-carotene, biotin, vitamin C, calcium, chlorine, magnesium, potassium, phosphorus, iron.	B vitamins, vitamin E, copper.	Sweet, delicious juice that is best for mixing, as this fruit yields little liquid. Antioxidant immune system booster that is good for cleansing the digestive tract and general detoxification.
Strawberry	Beta-carotene, folic acid, biotin, vitamins C and E, calcium, chlorine, magnesium, phosphorus, potassium.	B vitamins, iron, zinc.	Another delicious juice with a small yield. Antioxidant, cleansing, energizing, immune system booster.

Top 20 vegs for juicing

Vegetable	Rich in	Traces of	Benefits
Carrot	Beta-carotene, folic acid, vitamin C, calcium, magnesium, potassium.	B vitamins, iron, zinc.	Sweet, thick juice that is one of the most powerful antioxidants, detoxifiers and normalizers of the body. Particularly cleansing for the liver and intestines, it is also recommended for increasing energy, skin and eye problems, ulcers, and improving the milk of nursing mothers.
Beetroot	Beta-carotene, folic acid, vitamins B6 and C, calcium, iron, potassium.	B vitamins, zinc.	Sweet, purple juice that is one of the most powerful of the antioxidant immune system boosters. It helps to build up red blood cells and is profoundly detoxifying. Also believed to be helpful for anaemia, memory, concentration, menstrual and menopausal problems, and for stimulating the lymphatic and circulation systems.
Broccoli	Beta-carotene, folic acid, vitamin C, iron, potassium, sodium.	B vitamins, zinc.	Too strong on its own, but great mixed with carrot juice. Powerful antioxidant and energizer.
Cabbage	Beta-carotene, folic acid, calcium, potassium, and vitamins C and E.	B vitamins, iron, zinc.	Another bitter juice that needs to be mixed with something sweeter. A powerful antioxidant and cleanser that is beneficial for constipation, the skin and ulcers.
Tomato	Beta-carotene, biotin, folic acid, vitamins C and E, chlorine, calcium, magnesium, potassium, sodium.	B vitamins, sulphur, iron, zinc.	Delicious juice that is a cleansing, antioxidant, immune system booster. Energizing and good for the skin.
Watercress	Beta-carotene, vitamins C and E, calcium, iron, magnesium, sodium, potassium.	B vitamins, copper, zinc.	One of the most powerful antioxidants, with a strong, peppery taste – so dilute it well with a milder juice. Very cleansing and a great immune system booster, it is particularly good for anaemia, low blood pressure, increasing energy levels and protecting against disease.
Celery	Folic acid, vitamin C, calcium, manganese, potassium.	B vitamins, vitamin E.	Deliciously salty taste, which really perks up milder vegetable juices. Cleansing, cooling (in hot weather), calming juice, which helps to build red blood cells, lower high blood pressure and overcome fluid retention.
Lettuce	Beta-carotene, vitamin C, calcium, folic acid, phosphorus, potassium, sodium.	B vitamins, copper, iron, magnesium, zinc.	Most lettuces are quite bitter – Cos being the mildest tasting – so mix them with something sweeter. Antioxidant and very detoxifying, lettuce juice is very beneficial for the skin and is also very calming.
Peppers	Beta-carotene, folic acid, vitamin C, calcium, potassium, magnesium.	B vitamins, vitamin E, iron, zinc.	Yellow and red peppers are sweeter than green. Powerful antioxidants, immune system boosters and detoxifiers, good for recuperation, the skin, nails and hair.

Vegetable	Rich in	Traces of	Benefits
Spinach	Beta-carotene, vitamins B3 and C, folic acid, calcium, iron, potassium.	–	Peppery juice that should be used only in mixes and in moderation due to its oxalic acid content. Very powerful antioxidant and immune system booster. Cleansing for the whole body, particularly the digestive system. Also beneficial for teeth, gums, headaches and anaemia.
Turnip (and Swede)	Folic acid, vitamin C, calcium, magnesium, phosphorus, potassium.	B vitamins.	Peppery juice (especially turnip) with a very high calcium content which is particularly good for teeth and bones. Antioxidant, cleansing.
Cucumber	Beta-carotene, folic acid, vitamin C, calcium, potassium, silica.	B vitamins, iron, zinc.	High water content makes cucumber good for mixing with stronger juices. Very good for cleansing the whole system, it is the best diuretic juice available and excellent for rheumatism, high blood pressure and as a beauty boost for skin, hair and nails.
Chicory	Beta-carotene, folic acid, iron, potassium.	–	Like celery, the taste of chicory perks up blander juices. Antioxidant immune system booster.
Celeriac	Vitamin C, calcium, magnesium, phosphorus, potassium.	B vitamins, iron.	Nutty, delicious taste, good for mixing. Antioxidant, good for strengthening bones and teeth.
Onion	Folic acid, vitamin C, calcium, chlorine, magnesium, phosphorus, potassium.	B vitamins, copper, iron, zinc.	Not surprisingly, another very strong juice – use very sparingly for its great detoxifying, antioxidant, immune system boosting properties. Very good for respiratory ailments.
Fennel	Vitamin C, calcium, potassium.	Vitamin B6.	Its strong aniseed taste will perk up blander juices. A very cleansing juice, particularly for the liver and digestive system. Also a good diuretic.
Parsnip	B vitamins, calcium, folic acid, magnesium, phosphorus, potassium, sulphur, vitamins C and E.	Copper, iron, zinc.	Sweet-tasting juice, ideal for mixing with other root vegetables. Energizing, fortifying, particularly useful for bronchial and respiratory problems, and for brittle nails.
Garlic	Folic acid, vitamin C, calcium, iron, potassium.	B vitamins, zinc.	You need only a tiny amount of this juice (for obvious reasons), but it is a powerful antioxidant and immune system booster, which protects the heart and promotes circulation. It is anti-viral and kills parasites in the stomach and intestines.
Sweet potato	Beta-carotene, folic acid, vitamins C and E, calcium, chlorine, magnesium, phosphorus, potassium.	B vitamins, sodium, sulphur, iron.	Better-tasting than potato and more valuable nutritionally, this antioxidant immune system boosting juice is good for cellular protection.
Radish	Folic acid, vitamin C, calcium, iron, magnesium, potassium.	B vitamins, sodium, sulphur, zinc.	Strong peppery flavour, so use only a little in a mix. Powerful detoxifying, energizing antioxidant that is particularly good for respiratory infections (clears mucus).

Other **fruits and vegetables**

Fruit	Rich in	Traces of	Benefits
Blueberry	Beta-carotene, vitamin C, folic acid.	Iron, calcium, potassium.	Dark, sweet, thick juice, best diluted. Powerful immune system booster and antioxidant.
Cranberry	Beta-carotene, vitamin C, folic acid, calcium, magnesium, phosphorus, potassium.	B vitamins, copper, iron.	Far from sweet, so mix it with a sweeter juice and enjoy its tang. This immune system boosting antioxidant is useful for cystitis and urinary infections.
Fig	Beta-carotene, vitamin C, folic acid, calcium, iron, potassium.	–	Delicate flavour, good to mix with other juices. Immune system boosting antioxidant, useful for digestive cleansing.
Gooseberry	Beta-carotene, vitamin C, calcium, sulphur, magnesium, phosphorus, potassium.	B vitamins, vitamin E, iron, zinc.	Needs to be mixed with a sweeter juice. Antioxidant immune system booster.
Grapefruit	Beta-carotene, vitamin C, folic acid, calcium, magnesium, phosphorus, potassium, bioflavonoids.	B vitamins, vitamin E, iron, copper, manganese, zinc.	This should be mixed with a sweeter juice. Immunity booster, very cleansing, reduces cholesterol.
Guava	Beta-carotene, vitamin C, calcium, magnesium, phosphorus, potassium.	B vitamins, iron, zinc.	Thick, delicious juice, best mixed with others. Antioxidant, cleansing.
Lemon	Beta-carotene, vitamin C, calcium, magnesium, phosphorus, potassium, bioflavonoids.	B vitamins, iron.	Very bitter juice used to add zest to sweeter mixes. Good for fighting off infections, very cleansing, particularly for the kidneys and liver.
Lime	Beta-carotene, vitamin C, bioflavonoids, folic acid, calcium, phosphorus, potassium.	B vitamins, iron, zinc.	Very similar to lemon juice. Antioxidant, immune system booster.
Passion fruit	Beta-carotene, calcium, vitamins B3 and C, magnesium, phosphorus, potassium.	B vitamins, iron.	Sweet juice to mix with others. Antioxidant, very cleansing to the digestive tract.
Tangerine	Beta-carotene, calcium, folic acid, vitamin C, magnesium, phosphorus, potassium.	B vitamins, iron.	A sweeter version of orange juice. Antioxidant, immune system boosting, cleansing.

Vegetable	Rich in	Traces of	Benefits
Alfalfa	Beta-carotene, calcium, magnesium, phosphorus, potassium, silicon, vitamin B complex, C and E.	–	Not a particularly palatable juice, so mix this with something sweet (for example, carrot juice). Great antioxidant and immune system booster.
Beansprouts	B vitamins.	–	Again, this needs to be diluted with a sweeter juice. Its antioxidant and cleansing properties make the taste worthwhile.
Brussels sprouts	Beta-carotene, calcium, folic acid, vitamin C, magnesium, potassium.	B vitamins, zinc, iron.	Too strong to be drunk neat, dilute this with carrot juice. Another powerful antioxidant.
Cauliflower	Beta-carotene, calcium, folic acid, vitamin C, magnesium, phosphorus, potassium.	B vitamins, iron, zinc.	Mix with sweeter juices. Good antioxidant, cleanser.
Kale	Beta-carotene, calcium, iron, folic acid, sulphur, potassium, phosphorus, sodium, and vitamins B3 and C.	Vitamins B1 and B2.	Like all the dark green vegetables, kale is a strong-tasting juice that should be diluted with a milder one. Cleansing antioxidant immune system booster.
Leek	Beta-carotene, vitamin C, folic acid, biotin, calcium, chlorine, magnesium, phosphorus, potassium.	B and E vitamins, iron, zinc.	Onion-flavoured juice (but less strong than onion) with powerful antioxidant, energizing and immune system boosting properties. Good for arthritis and other inflammatory conditions. Soothing for the nervous system.
Potato	Vitamin C, folic acid, calcium, chlorine, potassium, sulphur, phosphorus.	B vitamins, iron, zinc.	Use only a small amount mixed with other juices. A deep-cleansing juice that is good for the nervous system and the skin.
Seaweed	Beta-carotene, vitamin B12, calcium, iodine, iron, magnesium, potassium, zinc.	–	Salty tasting and mineral-packed juice. Powerful detoxifier and energizer.

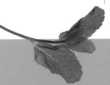

Herbs and spices

Herb or Spice	Rich in	Benefits
Chives	Beta-carotene, vitamin C, calcium, iron, zinc.	Peppery flavour, perks up other juices, and has many of the benefits of onion juice, to a somewhat reduced degree.
Ginger	Beta-carotene, vitamin C, calcium, iron, zinc, plus unique oils stimulating to the circulation.	This delicious, warming spice stimulates the circulation, relieves aches and pains, soothes nausea and indigestion, and relieves colds and sore throats.
Mint	Beta-carotene, vitamin C, calcium, iron.	A fresh flavour and a boost for the digestive system, it is cleansing and antioxidant.
Parsley	Beta-carotene, vitamin C, folic acid, calcium, iron, zinc, potassium.	Antioxidant, cleansing, calming: good for both digestive and nervous systems; diuretic: helpful for bladder or kidney conditions.

If you now feel convinced that fruit
and vegetable juices would have a positive
effect upon your health, your next step is plan-
ning just how you are going to incorporate them into
your diet. In fact, juicing is not at all mysterious. It is a
very simple process, and buying a juicer has never been
easier, with a wide variety of makes and models available in
most department stores, from the very inexpensive to costly

Introducing juices into your day

super-juicers. This section of the book takes you through the
whole process of choosing the right type of juicer for your
needs. Most importantly, it shows you what is suitable for
juicing (some of the fruit and vegetables listed here may
surprise you, but you'll find them delicious when you
try them), what to look for when you are buying
produce, how to prepare fruit and vegetables,
and even how to make real fruit ice lollies
for children.

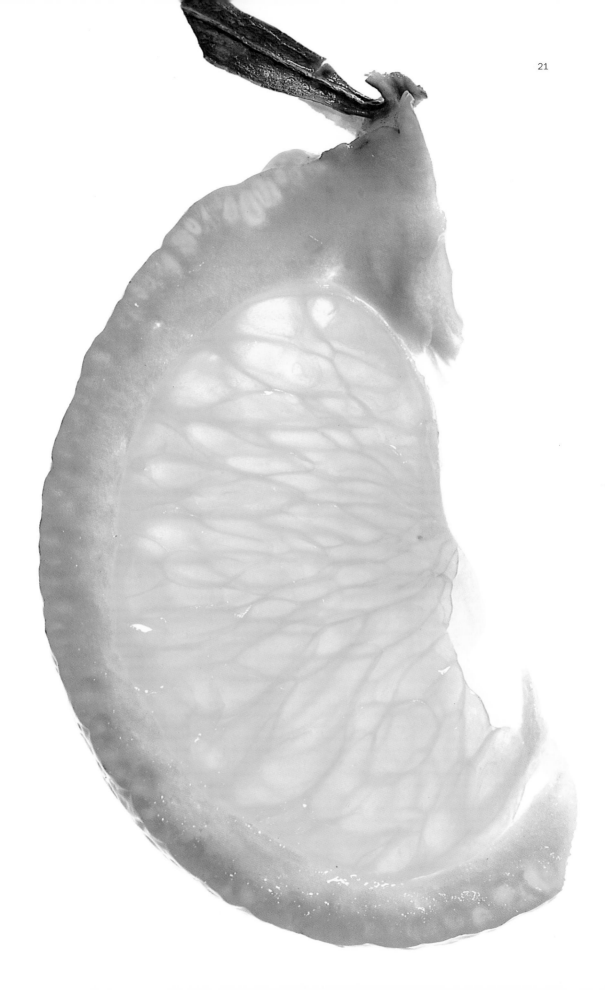

Home-made
juices

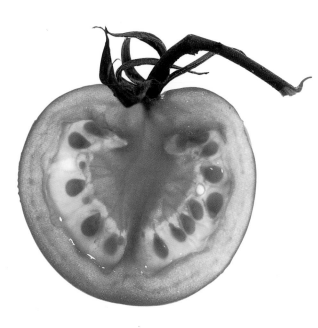

Juices you make yourself will bear little or no resemblance to those which you buy in supermarkets. This is true on several levels; what they look like, how they taste, and their nutritional value. Shop-bought juice is generally made from concentrates and contains various undesirable additives, including sugar and preservatives. If you do buy a carton of juice, always look for one that promises 100 per cent pure "fresh" juice, as opposed to the "long life" variety. Don't be fooled by the different types of exotic-looking "juice" drinks. These contain only a small proportion of fruit juice and their main ingredients are sugar and water.

There are a few honourable exceptions in the form of freshly squeezed juices – usually orange, apple or carrot – but juice is at the peak of its nutritional value at the moment it is made. After that, it gradually deteriorates and its goodness is lost. The juice you make yourself at home and drink immediately is therefore going to give you the greatest health benefits. Still, if you can buy a bottle of fresh carrot juice from the shop around the corner from your office, take advantage of it!

The other option, if you're out all day, is a juice bar. These are opening up in increasing numbers in towns all over Europe, the United States, Australia and New Zealand. They offer some delicious concoctions, many with added extras, such as spirulina, which have their own great health bonuses. Check the ingredients first before you decide which to buy; some may use dairy produce to make smoothies, or nuts (a problem if you suffer from allergies), while others may contain some ingredients that dieters would probably want to avoid, such as coconut milk. Juice bars are also a great source of inspiration for making your own juices, where you may well find new and interesting ingredients that you wouldn't otherwise think of trying.

Nothing will beat your home-made juice, though. It tastes wonderful and is much more nutritious than anything on the supermarket shelf. You should expect it to look rather different, however. You may be a bit surprised by its bright or murky colour, much thicker consistency or froth on top. Don't worry – this is how home-made juice is supposed to look. Just stir (don't strain) and drink it.

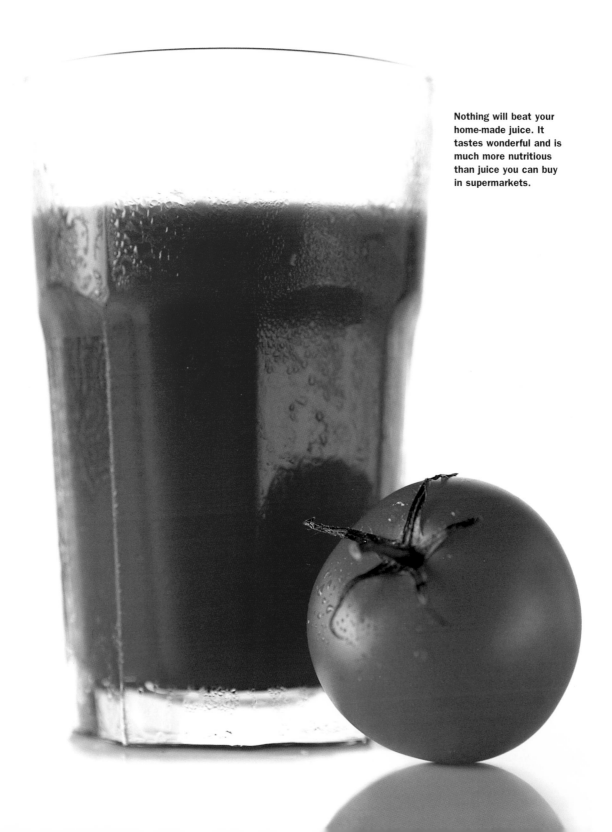

Nothing will beat your home-made juice. It tastes wonderful and is much more nutritious than juice you can buy in supermarkets.

Juicing
through the day

Drinking freshly made juices will bring you great health benefits in the long-term but, to begin with, you may find that they affect you more than you expected. This is partly because, since the juices are so cleansing, they tend to sweep your digestive system clean, so you may find yourself going to the lavatory more often than usual. Some juices cleanse the liver of toxic build-up or flush the kidneys so that their cleansing function improves. As the juices detoxify your body, you may experience some unwanted side effects, such as headaches or blemishes. Don't worry. These are all very much short-term problems and, as your body is cleansed and becomes more accustomed to fresh juices, these side effects will vanish.

To begin with, then, it is probably best to limit your intake to two glasses of juice a day. Ideally, one should be drunk early in the morning, at breakfast time, and the other at lunch time. If the latter is not possible, you can have the second juice in the early evening – provided that you choose one that does not have too stimulating an effect, which could interfere with your sleep. If your body can cope comfortably with two juices a day, you can go up to three immediately. If you have side effects, though, give yourself time to get used to the juices before increasing the quantity you drink.

Many people who are accustomed to juicing can drink six, or even eight, glasses of juice a day, especially when on a juice detoxification plan (see pages 100–123). On a regular basis, however, two or three large fresh juices every day are an ideal way to safeguard your health.

Each of the different juices in this book has a particular effect. Many of them can be used as part of a healing plan, in which case you may want to focus on a few specific types of juice. However, if you are juicing primarily as a means of boosting your immune system and general health, you should drink as wide a variety of different juices as possible. You do need to balance fruit with vegetable juices, however. Fruit juices are delicious, but tend to contain a lot of natural sugars (fructose) which could overload your system, so they should be alternated with vegetable juices.

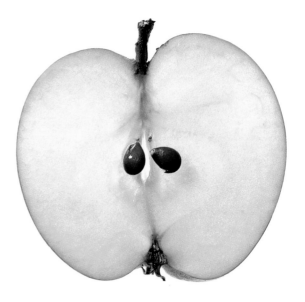

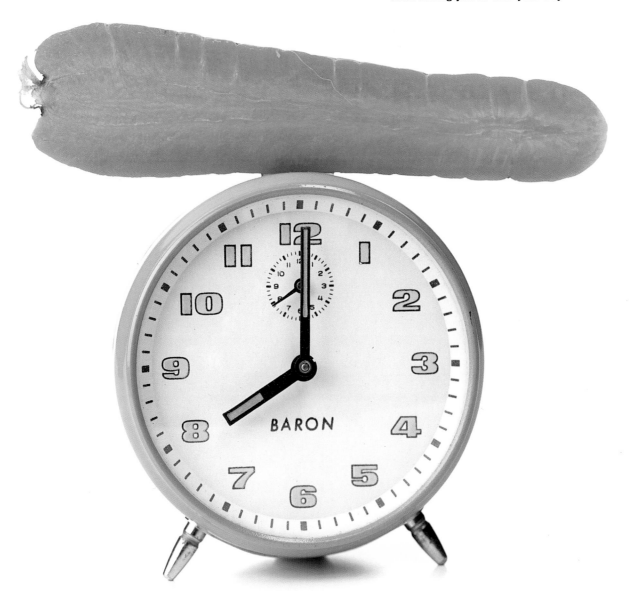

	If you drink three juices a day, follow this schedule for balancing them:
Breakfast	■ An ideal start for the day is a fruit-based juice, particularly one that contains an apple. This will cleanse your system and give you energy for the day ahead.
Lunch	■ A sweet, vegetable-based juice is a good pick-me-up in the middle of the day when energy can start to flag. One with carrot or beetroot as the basis of a mixture is stimulating for the whole body.
Evening	■ A dark-green vegetable juice is both healing and calming. Many such juices are great as blood cleansers and have a soothing effect upon the body.

What to juice
and add to juices

O nce you have bought a juicer and started experimenting, you will find the question is more what *not* to juice rather than what to juice. At the juice counter in the supermarket, there is little to choose from – usually only orange, grapefruit, apple, tomato and sometimes carrot. However, as you are about to find out, these shop-bought juices bear little resemblance to real home-made ones. Since even the "fresh" ones are usually a couple of days old, they will have lost much of their potency by the time you drink them.

Most fruits and vegetables can be juiced, however unlikely some of the candidates may seem at first glance. Even the most solid root vegetables, which look as if they can't have any juice in them, can in fact make surprisingly good juices.

You can also add fresh herbs and spices to concoctions for a whole new slant on nutrients and flavours. Fresh ginger, for example, is good in many drinks, particularly those containing apple. It is widely acknowledged to act as a stimulant, as well as warming the body.

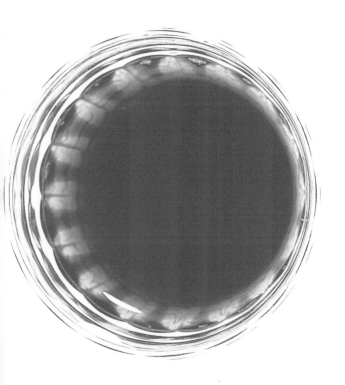

A FEW GOLDEN RULES FOR JUICING:

1 Juice vegetables and fruits separately – with the exception of apples and carrots, which mix with anything and cross all borders.

2 The darker the juice, the more it needs to be diluted. Be wary of drinking strong juices (like those made from watercress) by themselves. Strong flavours should be diluted with water or mixed with other juices, such as carrot or cucumber. Also, always dilute juices with water for young children (see page 85).

3 Always try to buy organic produce, so that you can use the whole fruit or vegetable, including leaves, stalks and roots.

4 Whenever possible, scrub the surface of the fruit and vegetables rather than peel them.

5 Vary juices so that you consume a wide range of fruits and vegetables. Advice about when to drink fruit or vegetable juice may be found on page 24.

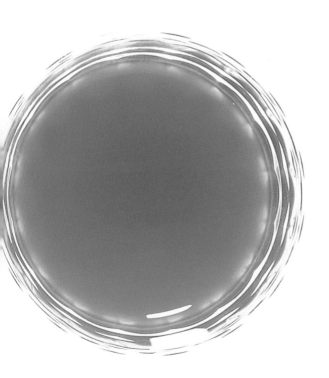
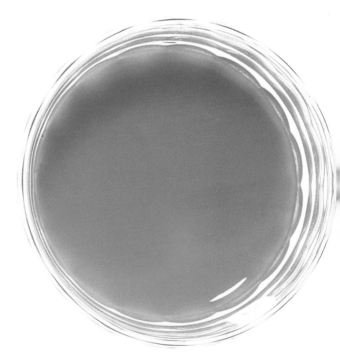

Only the **best**

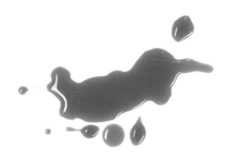

When you go to your local market to buy fruit and vegetables for juicing, remember one simple rule. Buy the best. Don't be tempted, because it's for drinking from a glass rather than being presented on a plate, to go for produce that is obviously past its sell-by date. The better the condition of the raw materials you use, the better the nutritional value of your juice – not to mention its taste.

In general, it is always advisable to buy fruit and vegetables that are in season. This way, you know that they have not been forced to fruit early, which usually means that they have been over-fed fertilizers and been through some pretty unnatural growing conditions. The same thing happens to baby versions of some vegetables, like corn. Of course, if you live in a cool, northern climate, some fruits (such as bananas and mangoes) will never be in season,

as they won't grow in your part of the world. If they must travel a long way, they may well be subject to long-term refrigeration or be picked long before they are ripe in order to survive the journey. Because the flavours are so delicious, they are too good to miss altogether. Choose carefully and look for produce that is not too hard or pale.

As a general rule, look for fruit that is ripe, but not overripe. When fruit is at the peak of its maturity, it will be particularly potent nutritionally and will also yield the most juice. Ripe fruits are also easier on the digestive system. Avoid anything bruised or wilted, or anything that has lost its bloom through sitting on a shelf for too long. If fruit is not obviously freshly picked, go for produce that is kept at least semi-refrigerated.

When choosing vegetables, it is important that they should be in as complete a state as

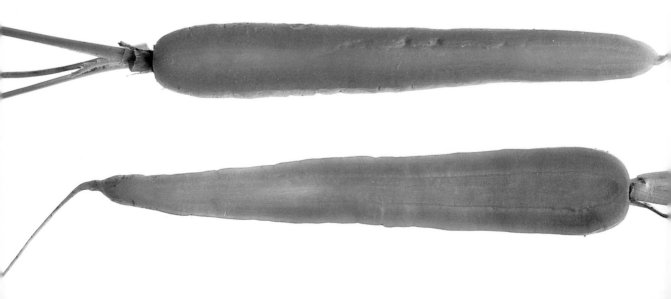

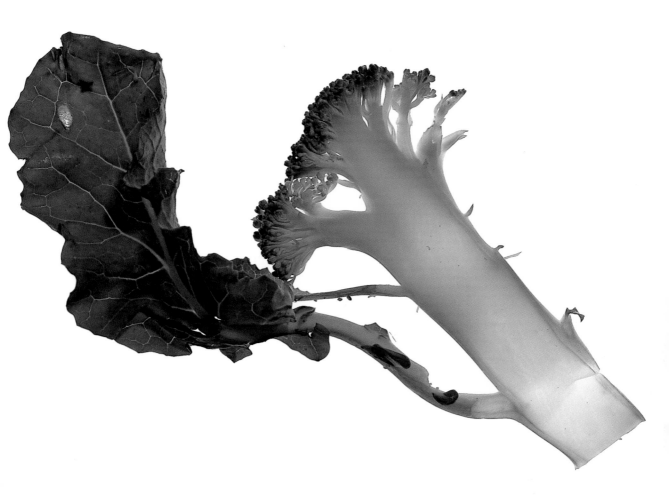

possible. This is because you can juice their outer leaves – actually often the most nutritious part (along with the stalks and roots) – provided that the vegetables are grown organically (see pages 30–31).

Look for the freshest vegetables possible, or grow your own if you have a garden. This will ensure peak freshness as you can juice as soon as you have picked them. There are also a great many farms and market gardens where you can buy produce direct, so again you will be getting just-picked produce. Indeed, you can pick your own fruit and vegetables on some farms, and save yourself some money, too.

There is also an increasingly widely available service of delivering organic fruit and vegetables direct to your home. This can be quite good fun if you opt for a mixed box of produce every week, whose contents depend on what the delivery company has decided are the best buys. This way, you get a surprise when you open the box!

WHAT YOU CAN'T JUICE

There are some things that just won't juice, no matter how good your juicer may be. Their juice content cannot be separated from their pulp and so you get either very little juice or a sort of sludge at the bottom of a cup! However, some (banana and pawpaw are examples) are worth putting through your juicer anyway for the simple reason that their flavours are so wonderful. Give them a good stir as you drink them in order to keep them mixed. Other fruits, though, such as avocado, are really not worth the effort; it's better just to eat them!

Why **organic?**

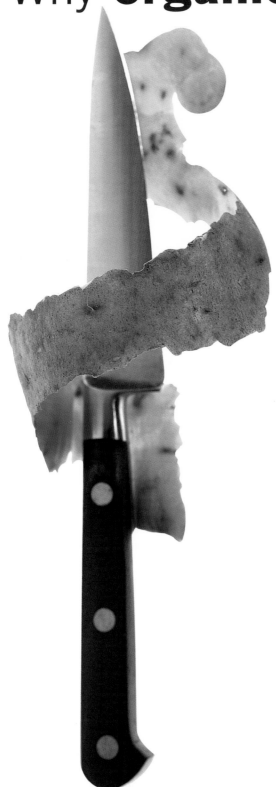

Besides buying fruit and vegetables that are at the peak of their nutritional value, it is also important, if possible, to buy organic ones. There is, of course, a great deal of controversy about whether the levels of farming chemicals found in food can damage health, and government regulations stipulate acceptable levels for safety reasons. However, significantly higher chemical residue levels have been found in food samples, and this is obviously very worrying.

In the UK in March 1997, for instance, the British Ministry of Agriculture discovered that organophosphate and pesticide residue levels in apples and peaches exceeded their safety guidelines, and officially advised that all fruit given to children should be peeled before consumption. However, peeling does not remove systemic pesticides, which are absorbed into the entire fruit.

CHEMICAL AND GM DANGERS

Moreover, if high levels of particular chemicals are dangerous, even low levels can hardly be good for people; so it is not unreasonable to try to avoid them altogether. Tests in which volunteers were exposed to the apple pesticide triazophos, for instance, resulted in headaches, diarrhoea, stomach cramps and had detrimental effects on blood plasma, which continued for up to four weeks. Furthermore, different chemicals are often used on the same crop, which results in a cocktail of effects, which may increase toxicity. This could be a problem for people who eat fruit and vegetables.

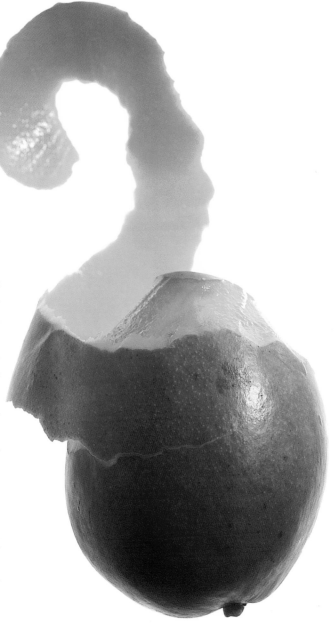

One of the most worrying trends these days is the extensive use of nitrate fertilizers. Nitrates are not dangerous until they react with other chemicals to form nitrite. If nitrate is converted to nitrite within the human digestive tract, it may go on to form carcinogenic (cancer-producing) nitrosamines. Excessive levels of nitrate can cause nitrate cyanosis (often called "blue baby syndrome"), which occurs in babies under six months old. Nitrate levels are particularly high in intensively farmed vegetables.

In the meantime, more new fertilizers, pesticides and weedkillers are appearing on the market. Most worryingly, it is virtually impossible to carry out tests on their long-term effects before they have already arrived in our food.

The same concerns are felt even more strongly about genetically modified foods. There is widespread feeling that there has not been sufficient time to evaluate the possible long-term effects on agriculture and food production, or even on nature itself, and that, once let loose in the agricultural world, it will be impossible to put this particular genie back into its bottle.

BETTER NUTRITIONAL VALUE

Apart from the risks involved in eating non-organic produce, evidence is growing that there is more vital nutritional value in organic fruit and vegetables. Over thirty studies have shown that levels of important individual nutrients like vitamin C and zinc are generally higher in organic produce.

Farming methods are not the only problem. The heavy metal content of vehicle exhaust fumes can also contaminate produce. So never buy produce that is sold beside a busy road.

Finally, there is one more good reason to buy organic food. Apart from questions concerning health and the nutritional value of food, there is also the indisputable fact that most people find organic fruit and vegetables more full of flavour and, quite simply, delicious.

Juicing is the
simplest of processes,
and you can juice almost all
fruit and vegetables. You must,
however, have a proper juicer. You
can't make do with a food processor, unless
it has a special juicing attachment. Other than that,
the only equipment you will need is a sharp knife and a

How
to juice

chopping board. Preparing your fruit and vegetables is also very straight-
forward, and basically consists of cutting them down into the right-sized
chunks to fit into your juicer. Certain parts, for example, stones, kernels
or very hard outer skins, should be discarded, but generally fruit
and vegetables, provided they are organic and thoroughly
cleaned, should be juiced in as whole a state as possible.

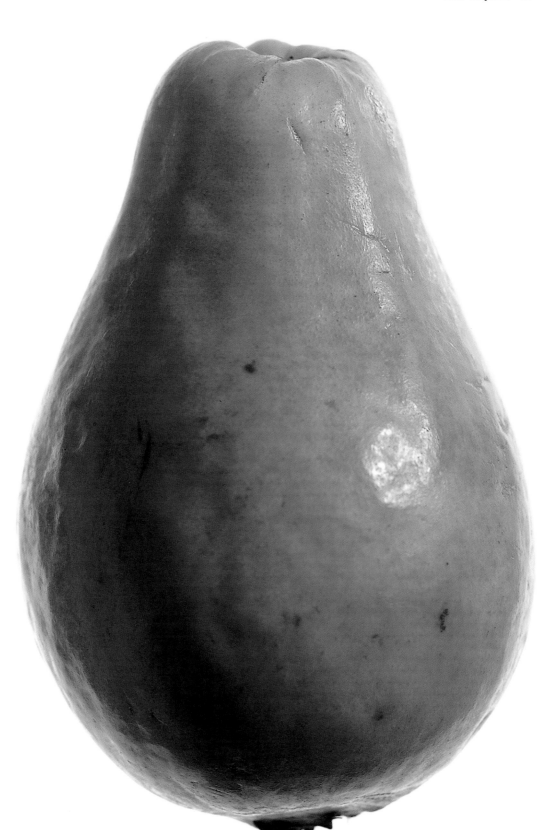

Choosing
a juicer

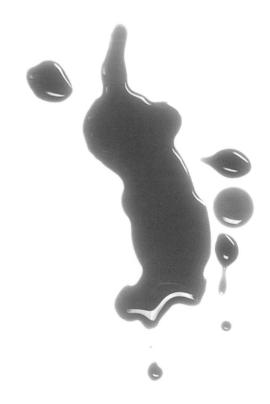

Juicers are becoming an increasingly familiar sight in kitchens these days as many people, tempted by what they have tasted in a juice bar or found on the fresh juice shelf at the supermarket, have decided to make their own juices at home.

The only thing you must remember when juicing at home is that you have to use a proper juicer. You can't make juice in a food processor or liquidizer, because only a juicer will separate juice from pulp. It is possible to make juice by hand, but it is such a time-consuming and messy process, involving endless grating and pressing of pulp through a sieve that, frankly, it's just not worth the effort.

Juicers are now cheaper and more widely available than ever. Here are the options:

1 Citrus juicer. This is the simplest and cheapest form of juicer and in its plainest form – as a lemon-squeezer – just about every kitchen has one already. There are glass versions where you just press the juice by hand against a central cone, and there are also electric versions that work on the same principle. These can, of course, be used only for citrus fruits, such as lemons, oranges, limes and grapefruit. However, only a small quantity of citrus juice is recommended for the body, because its acidic nature can be rather abrasive upon the digestive system.

You can juice citrus fruit in any of the other forms of juicer listed, but it is important to remember to remove as much of the peel and pith as possible.

2 Centrifugal juicer. The most compact, widely available and cheapest juicers work by centrifugal force. Fruit and vegetables are fed into a rapidly spinning grater which separates pulp (retained in the body of the machine) from juice (which runs into a separate jug). Juicing experts claim that centrifugal juicers supply fewer nutrients than masticating juicers (see below), although this has never been proven. What is true, though, is that centrifugal juicers produce slightly less juice than masticating ones.

3 Masticating juicer. This juicer mashes the fruit or vegetable and pushes it with great force through a mesh wire, thus producing a great quantity of juice. It tends to be more expensive than a centrifugal juicer.

4 Hydraulic press. This juicer extracts juice simply by exerting tremendous pressure on the fruit or vegetable. The juice is filtered out through mesh or muslin – efficient but expensive.

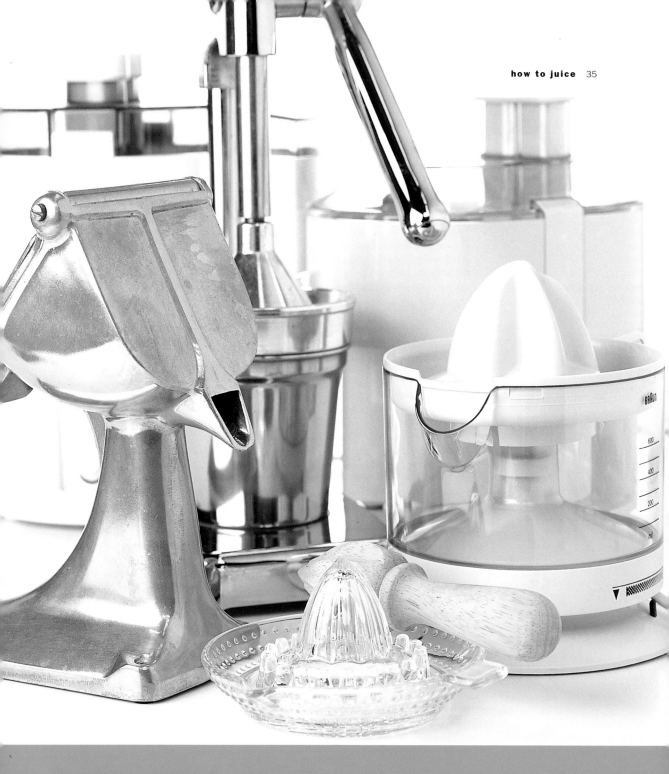

CLEANING THE JUICER

One of the most important things to consider when choosing a juicer is whether it can be taken apart and assembled easily – so check all of the models available in your price range from this point of view. If taking it apart and being able to clean it easily is impossible, you are hardly likely to use it regularly, because using it will simply become too much of a chore. Make sure that you can get into all of its corners to clean it, because pulp can be hard to dislodge.

If you buy a smaller juicer, bear in mind, also, that, if you want to make a large quantity of juice, you may need to empty and clean the juicer halfway through the juicing, as the machine will become clogged with pulp.

Preparing
produce

As has been suggested, it is always preferable to buy organic fruit and vegetables if you possibly can. Pesticides, fertilizers and herbicides really are to be avoided when what you ultimately want is the cleansing and detoxifying effect of pure fresh juice. Unfortunately, organic produce is far from available universally, but generally it is best, given the choice, to buy organic food whenever you can.

You will need to clean any fruit and vegetables you use very thoroughly, as, with few exceptions, you don't peel when juicing. If you buy organic produce, use all the leaves and green tops, too. Peeling loses the enzymes, minerals and vitamins that are just below the surface of the skin of the fruit and vegetables, and you want to preserve these at all costs.

WASHING FRUIT AND VEGETABLES

If you are using organic produce, you should wash thoroughly in warm water all fruit and vegetables which will be juiced with their skins. If you are using non-organic produce, wash it in warm water with a little washing-up liquid added to it, then rinse it thoroughly in fresh, cold water. If there is a lot of dirt on the fruit and vegetables, or their surfaces are rough, use a clean brush to scrub them gently.

CHOPPING UP THE PRODUCE

You will need a sharp knife – very sharp in the case of tough root vegetables – and a chopping board. Cut the fresh produce into chunks as large as your juicer can process. However, only start cutting when you are ready to juice; this way, your fruits and vegetables will oxidize as little as possible, and fewer vital nutrients will be lost to the air.

HOLISTIC JUICING

When juicing, you should include as much of the fruit or vegetable as possible, if it is organic. However, if it is not organic, don't include leaves, roots or the tops.

If the produce is organic, everything can go into the juicer. This includes the peel of most fruits and vegetables, but excludes very tough exteriors, such as those of melons, pineapples, bananas, mangoes, pawpaws, oranges and lemons. Pips from apples, oranges, grapes and pears and so on may go into the juicer, but stones from apricots, plums, peaches, cherries and mangoes should not. Most seeds are juicable including those in melon or watermelons but pawpaw seeds should be discarded before juicing. Pick the stalks off grapes, berries or currants before you juice them, although as long as they are not too woody, you needn't be too fussy.

The outer leaves of vegetables like cabbage and lettuce can be juiced also. In fact, these often have the highest proportion of nutrients.

Always leave the outer peel on vegetables (just give them a good scrub), unless they have been waxed – as cucumbers often are, for instance. Papery peels – such as those of onions and garlic – should, however, be completely removed.

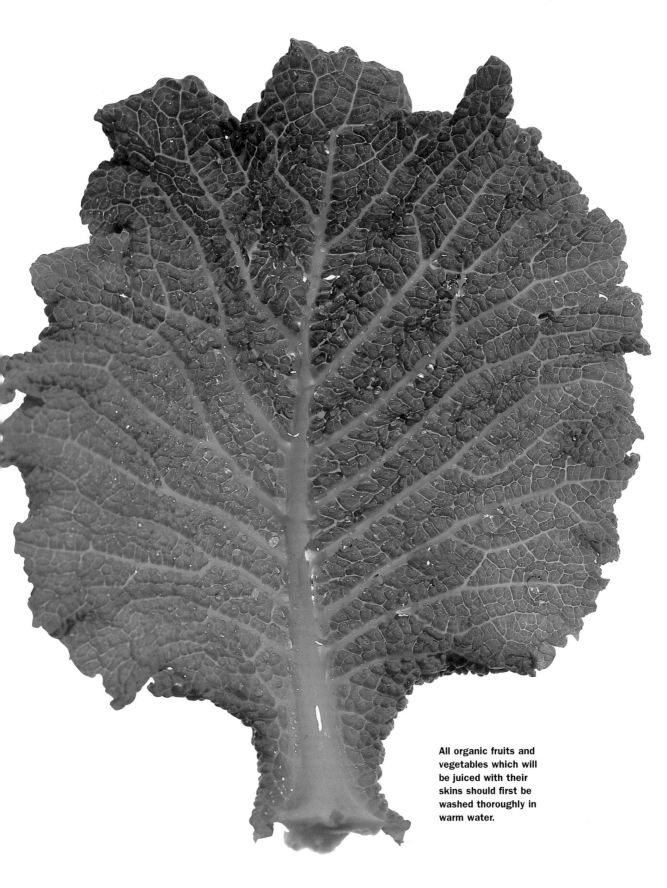

All organic fruits and vegetables which will be juiced with their skins should first be washed thoroughly in warm water.

Storing
produce and juice

A lways use your fruit and vegetables as soon as you can. The fresher the produce, the fresher and more nutritious the juice. Before you juice, keep all ripe ingredients (with the exception of bananas, which will quickly turn black) in your refrigerator. If fruit or vegetables aren't ripe, leave them at room temperature to ripen them a little further, but keep a very close watch on them (especially any organic ones) as they can start to go mouldy very quickly.

If you can, use herbs and sprouts that are still growing in their containers when you buy them. They can then grow and generate nutrients right up until the minute you use them.

The same, of course, is true if you have a vegetable or fruit garden. For the ultimate in freshness, pick produce the moment you are ready to juice it.

As soon as you cut into a fruit or vegetable and it becomes exposed to the air, oxidization takes place. This is the process that turns an apple brown when you cut it in half, and during oxidization the fruit or vegetable loses vital nutrients. So, one of the rules of juicing is that you cut things up only when you are ready to use them, and that you then use, whenever possible, the whole fruit or vegetable, rather than store what is left over. With bigger ingredients – such as melons, pineapples and watermelons, it is unlikely that you will need to use the whole of the fruit unless you are making juice for lots of people. Where you use only a portion of a large fruit, such as a watermelon, you should seal the remainder tightly with cling film and store it in your refrigerator until you are ready to use the rest.

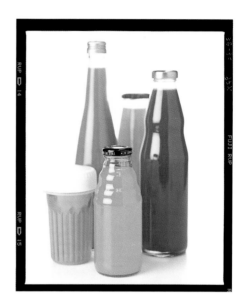

STORING JUICES

Oxidization also takes place after juicing, so another golden rule is to drink your juice the moment you have made it. However, if you are away from home and want to take juice with you to drink during the day, you can store it in a vacuum flask or a screw-topped glass bottle which you can then store in a refrigerator. You will lose some nutrients this way, but it's obviously better than having no juice at all. If the juice contains a mixture of ingredients, they are very likely to separate during the day, so stir it well to mix them all back together again.

If you are at home and have a juicer, it is better to make juice fresh as you need it, rather than to juice in bulk and store liquids in a refrigerator. Make different mixtures during the day, which is more beneficial in health terms (unless you are using a particular juice to relieve a specific ailment), as well as being more interesting.

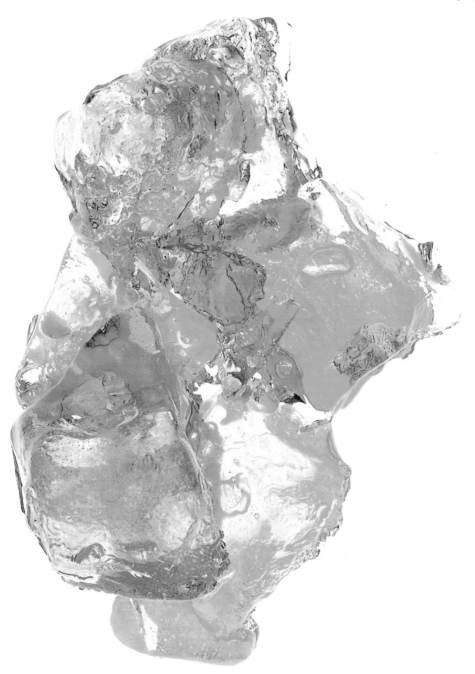

FREEZING JUICES

You can freeze juices, which is particularly useful if you have a glut of tomatoes or carrots in your vegetable garden. It is best to use single fruits or vegetables for freezing, as mixes can separate and do not freeze well.

Frozen juice is the ideal ice lolly for children, too. Lolly moulds are widely available in department stores nowadays. However, when you make lollies yourself, you know that they not only have no additives, but actually have positive health benefits.

Juicing
practicalities

There are a few practicalities to bear in mind when juicing. When making the juice itself, your machine (especially if it is one of the smaller, centrifugal kinds) will be able to process some kinds of fruit and vegetables more easily than others. The most difficult to liquidize are dense root vegetables (like turnips, swedes and potatoes), fibrous green vegetables (such as watercress, spinach and cabbage), and herbs. The best way to deal with this problem is to feed in only small quantities at a time and alternate them with a vegetable (such as carrot, celery or cucumber) which juices very easily and also cleans the juicer on the way.

No vegetables that are difficult to juice should ever be consumed on their own. Because their flavours are so strong, you should mix them with other things. This is important to consider when you begin to invent your own juices.

I will always remember the first time I made watercress juice. I was especially looking forward to trying it as a juice since watercress is something of which I am particularly fond. Of course, when I tried it neat, it brought tears to my eyes and made me gasp! Because of this, it is not a juice that I recommend on its own.

DILUTING JUICES

Generally, you can resolve the problem of very strong flavours by mixing them with sweeter, milder ones. However, there are some circumstances when you will want to dilute juices with water. Young children, the elderly, or those convalescing after illness, should not be given strong, undiluted juices. In these cases, dilute to taste with filtered or still, bottled water and, if the drinker prefers more sweetness, stir in a spoonful of organic honey.

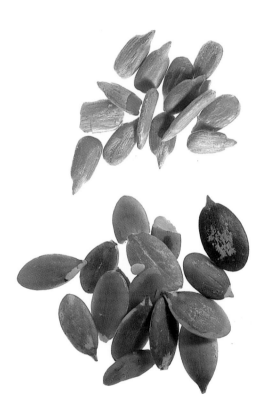

ADDED EXTRAS

As you become more experienced at juicing, you may want to add herbs and spices for their flavours or other properties. Ginger, for instance, has a very warming quality and is known to soothe respiratory ailments and make you feel warmer and more comfortable

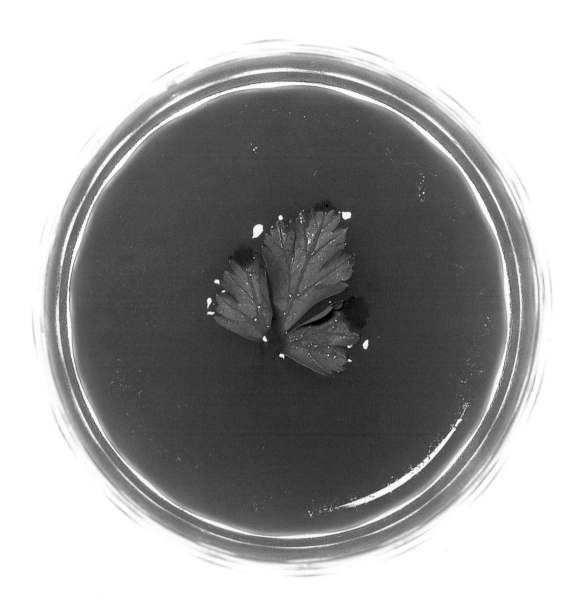

when you're feeling unwell. There are a number of ingredients that you can sprinkle on top of juices, particularly vegetable ones. These include spirulina, available in health shops, which contains a storehouse of vitamins (especially beta-carotene), minerals (especially iron), enzymes, carotenes, amino acids as well as other vital nutrients.

In addition, various seeds go well with vegetable juices, including sesame and cumin, and also wheatgerm. You can toast sesame seeds and wheatgerm to bring out their flavour.

SMOOTHIES

Finally, you can use juices to make smoothies. Fruit juices are best for this and the easiest way to make a smoothie is to juice or liquidize a few of your favourite fruits and mix them with a natural, organic yogurt in a food processor. The yogurt will obviously dilute the flavour of the fruit, so you will need to experiment to achieve the balance you prefer. You can add honey if you like a sweeter taste, or banana, which also sweetens, and will make the smoothie thicker.

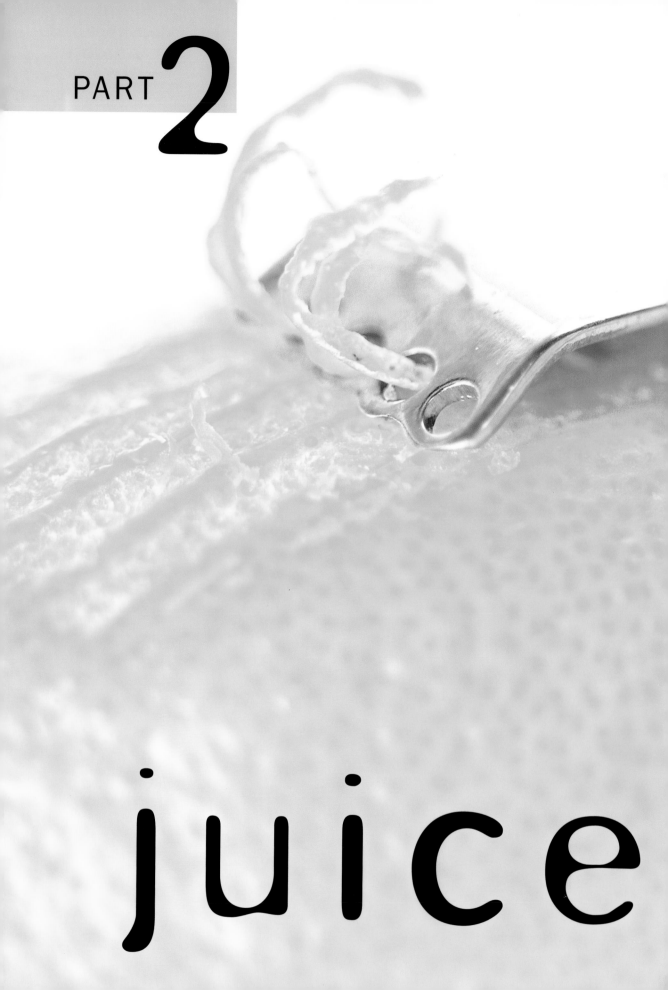

PART **2**

juice

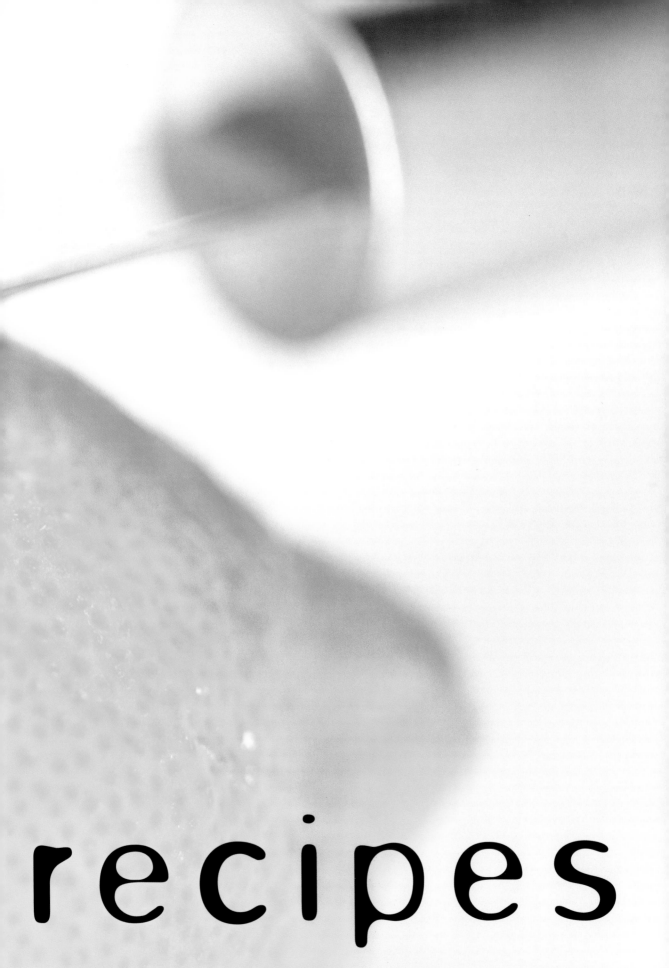

recipes

The recipes in this section of the
book are divided into two parts: fruit, and
vegetables. Vegetable juices tend to contain more powerful antioxidants with cancer-fighting qualities and are deeply
cleansing and revitalizing for the blood, major organs and the
digestive tract. Some vegetables – notably anything in the onion family,
and most green ones – have a very strong taste and should not be drunk neat,
but mixed with sweeter vegetable juices from carrot, beetroot and tomato. Fruit

100 recipes

juices, which taste wonderful and appeal especially to children, are very energizing a
they contain natural fruit sugars. However, constantly drinking fruit juices can upse
your blood sugar balance, so you should alternate them with vegetable juices. One
glass each morning is the minimum daily intake for an all-round immune system
booster and general health protection. Once accustomed to drinking fresh
juices, you can increase the number to four, or, if you are detoxifying,
six. You may feel that you need more fresh juices when you are
tired, under stress or convalescing. Keep your juicer on your
kitchen counter to remind you that you have a ready
source of vital nutrients at your fingertips.

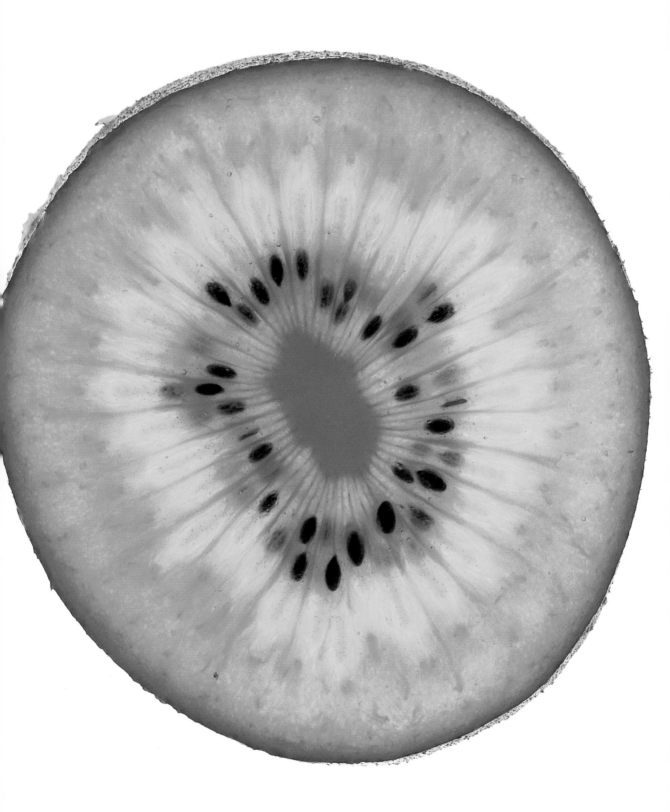

Fruit

Apple

STRAIGHT APPLE JUICE

Freshly-made apple juice is delicious, and much better than commercial juices. It has a lovely sweet flavour and you can mix it with just about any other fruit or vegetable. Full of antioxidants to protect the body against infection and boost the immune system, it is an excellent detoxifier (particularly of the digestive tract), laxative and diuretic. Apple juice reduces cholesterol, is good for various forms of inflammation (including gout, rheumatism and pulmonary conditions), provides extra energy and softens the skin.

3 apples

■ Wash and juice the apples, including the pips. Drink the juice immediately.
Rich in beta-carotene, folic acid, vitamin C, calcium, magnesium, pectin, phosphorus and potassium.
Traces of B vitamins, vitamin E, copper and zinc.

APPLE, PINEAPPLE AND GINGER

This thick, creamy, yellow juice is a wonderful combination of sweetness with the warming spicy taste of ginger. Ginger is very stimulating for the circulation, and simultaneously soothes nausea and menstrual cramps. Pineapple is very cleansing and a useful healer, while apple is, of course, a great cleanser and general

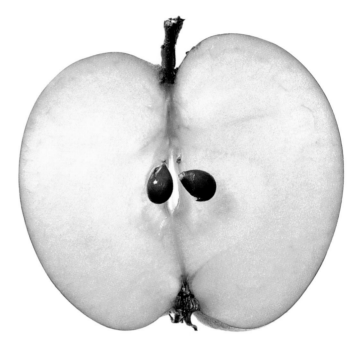

tonic. Therefore, this juice contains plenty of restorative power if you're feeling unwell.

½ inch ginger root
½ apple
⅓ large pineapple

■ Peel the ginger and pineapple. Wash the apple. Cut it and the pineapple into juiceable slices. Juice the ginger first, then the fruit. Stir in the froth and drink immediately.
Rich in beta-carotene, vitamin C, folic acid, pectin, calcium, magnesium, phosphorus, potassium and bromelian.
Traces of B vitamins, vitamin E, copper, iron and zinc.

APPLE, ORANGE AND PINEAPPLE

This is a lovely, sweet juice that is packed full of antioxidants. It is very cleansing and immune

system boosting, as well as extremely energizing. Considered to be an active cancer-fighting juice, it is also very good for the digestive system.

2 apples
¼ pineapple
Small bunch of green grapes
2 oranges

■ Remove the skin from the oranges and pineapple with a peeler or knife, wash the apples and grapes, removing the grapes from their stalk. Chop the fruit into sizes that will fit in your juicer, juice them and drink immediately.
Rich in beta-carotene, folic acid, vitamin C, calcium, magnesium, pectin, phosphorus, potassium and iron.
Traces of B vitamins, vitamin E, copper and zinc.

Blackberry

Blackberries are packed with nutrients, but produce only a small amount of juice, so must be mixed with other fruits that have a naturally higher water content. The small amount of juice they do produce, however, is really powerful stuff, being a general tonic and cleanser, as well as a powerful immune system booster that is considered to be particularly effective against respiratory ailments and anaemia.

■ BLACKBERRY AND WATERMELON

This is a dark, sweet, thick juice. It's an immune system booster, antioxidant, laxative and is a great energizer.

1 punnet of blackberries
⅙ watermelon
1 apple
1 banana

■ Wash the blackberries, and wash and chop up the apple.

Peel the watermelon, but keep the seeds. Cut the fruit into slices for juicing. Peel the banana. Juice in this order: banana, watermelon, blackberries, apple. Stir and drink the juice immediately.

Rich in beta-carotene, folic acid, pectin, calcium, magnesium, phosphorus, potassium, sodium, and vitamins B5, C, E and K.

Traces of other B vitamins, iron, copper and zinc.

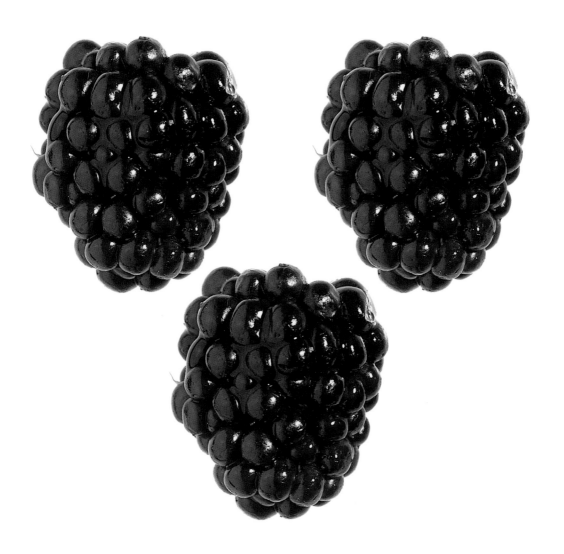

Pear

STRAIGHT PEAR JUICE

Pears produce a powerfully cleansing and health-building juice that gives you a surge of energy as well. Its high iodine content aids thyroid function, and it is both diuretic and slightly laxative. Pear juice is deliciously sweet and has one of the strongest and most evocative smells of all the fruits when juiced. The most important factor in making the best pear juice is that the pears used must be really ripe. Hard pears produce juice that is less sweet, and there will be a lot less liquid.

3 pears

■ Wash the pears, cut in half and juice them (including pips). Drink the juice immediately.
Rich in beta-carotene, folic acid, vitamin C, pectin, calcium, magnesium, phosphorus and potassium.
Traces of B vitamins, iron, copper, manganese and zinc.

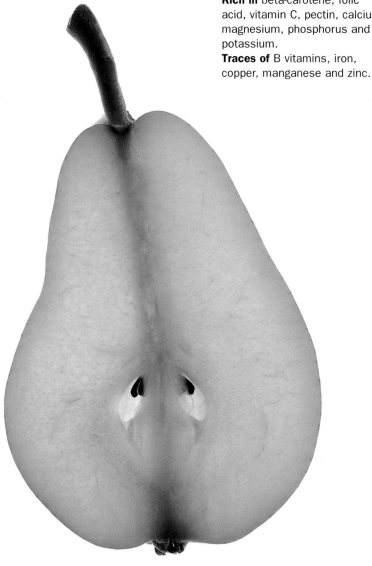

PEAR AND BANANA

This is a particularly beneficial juice when you're feeling tired or under stress. Both pears and bananas have an energizing effect on the body. This makes it a good breakfast drink too.

3 pears
1 banana

■ Peel and juice the banana. Discard the stalks from the pears, wash, cut and juice them. Stir and drink the juice immediately.
Rich in beta-carotene, folic acid, iodine, calcium, pectin, magnesium, phosphorus, potassium and vitamin C.
Traces of vitamins B, E, iron, manganese, copper and zinc.

PEAR AND PINEAPPLE

This is a sweet (depending on the ripeness of the fruit), pale yellow, creamy juice that is a very powerful cleanser. Pineapple contains bromelian, which not only stimulates the digestive system but actually removes bacteria and parasites, while pears act upon the intestines to sweep out toxins.

2 pears
¼ pineapple

■ Wash the pears and remove the peel from the pineapple. Cut both into suitably-sized chunks for juicing. Stir and drink the juice immediately.
Rich in beta-carotene, folic acid, vitamin C, pectin, bromelian, calcium, magnesium, phosphorus and potassium.
Traces of vitamins B and E, iron, copper, manganese and zinc.

Blackcurrants

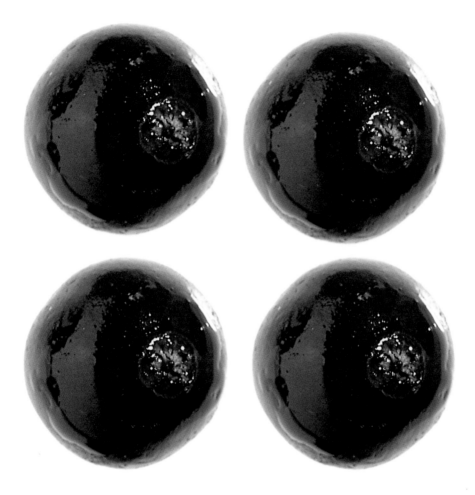

Blackcurrants are powerful antioxidants, but they yield very little juice and have an extremely strong taste, so they must be mixed with something sweet and juicy. They are well worth using with other juices, as they are highly antioxidant and are also said to protect the body against infection and certain forms of cancer. Blackcurrants also act as a cleanser of the blood and general energizer.

■ ALL-CURRANT COCKTAIL

A good all-round protective and energizing juice, this is very strongly flavoured, rich and sweet, with a slightly bitter aftertaste. Add another apple or banana if you prefer more sweetness.

1 punnet of blackcurrants
1 punnet of redcurrants
1 banana
1 apple

■ Wash the currants and remove them from their stalks. Juice the currants first, then peel the banana and add it to your mixture. Finally, wash and juice the apple. Stir and drink this combination immediately.
Rich in beta-carotene, folic acid, calcium, magnesium, phosphorus, potassium and vitamins C and E.
Traces of B vitamins, copper, iron and zinc.

Apricot

▍STRAIGHT APRICOT
▍JUICE

Like peaches and nectarines, apricots yield only small amounts of a thick, sweet, highly fragrant and delicious juice. It is full of nutrients, however, and is a marvellous antioxidant and energizer. It is also mildly laxative and beneficial for relieving PMS and menstrual cramps.

3–4 apricots

■ Wash and cut the apricots in half and remove their stones. Juice and drink immediately.
Rich in beta-carotene, folic acid, calcium, magnesium, iron, potassium, and vitamins C, B3 and B5.
Traces of copper and vitamins B1, B2 and B6.

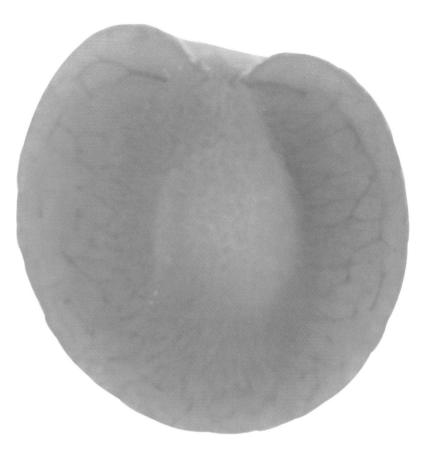

▍APRICOT AND
▍KIWI

Since apricots yield only a small amount of liquid, their juice is best consumed when mixed with the juice of another fruit. Adding kiwi is a great way to dilute the thick, rich apricot, and also adds another powerful energizing and detoxifying level to the juice. If possible, juice the kiwi leaving the skin on, since it contains many valuable nutrients. The skin also gives the juice a peppery, bitter taste. Peel the kiwi if you find this unpalatable. Apricot and kiwi is a great immune system booster and is said to be beneficial for the digestive system, as well as having laxative properties.

4 apricots
1 kiwi

■ Wash the ingredients and stone the apricots. Peel the kiwi if you prefer, then juice, stir and drink immediately.
Rich in beta-carotene, folic acid, calcium, magnesium, iron, potassium, phosphorus, bioflavonoids and vitamins C, B3 and B5.
Traces of copper, iron and vitamins B1, B2 and B6.

▍APRICOT AND
▍PINEAPPLE

This is a deliciously sweet juice. Full of protective antioxidants, it is gently cleansing to the digestive system. Said to have cancer-fighting properties, this juice is also beneficial for fighting colds.

4 apricots
½ pineapple
1 lemon

■ Peel the pineapple and lemon. Wash the apricots thoroughly and remove their stones. Juice the fruit. Drink immediately.
Rich in beta-carotene, folic acid, bromelian, calcium, magnesium, phosphorus, iron, potassium and vitamins B3, B5 and C.
Traces of other B vitamins, copper and zinc.

Pawpaw

▌STRAIGHT PAWPAW ▌JUICE

Pawpaws, or papayas, are probably my favourite fruits, and when my son and I lived in Polynesia, we had one every morning for breakfast during their season. Apart from being a delicious start to the day, one of the visible effects of this was that, for the first time in my life, I developed long, strong nails. Pawpaws are potent detoxifiers and very soothing to the digestive system. They are also said to protect the body from cancer. Pawpaw juice is fragrant and absolutely delicious, but probably a bit too thick to drink without mixing anything else with it – unless you use a spoon! Be very careful when handling pawpaws, as their skin and seeds can cause itching; wash your hands and never touch your eyes after handling pawpaws. It is one of the few fruits from which I would recommend removing the seeds. If you have a powerful juicer, you can include the skin; if not, peel the fruit and juice.

2 pawpaws

■ Peel or wash and cut the fruits in half, then scoop out the seeds. Cut them into chunks, juice and drink immediately.
Rich in beta-carotene, vitamin C, calcium, papain, phosphorus, flavonoids, magnesium and potassium.
Traces of B vitamins, iron, zinc.

▌PAWPAW AND ▌GINGER

This is not only a deliciously spicy juice; it also boosts the immune system and is said to fight cancer and the effects of ageing. To increase these effects still further, add some ginseng to the cocktail.

2 pawpaws
½ inch ginger root

■ Peel or wash the pawpaws and scoop out their seeds. Scrub the ginger. Juice and drink immediately.
Rich in beta-carotene, vitamin C, calcium, magnesium, phosphorus, potassium, papain and flavonoids.
Traces of B vitamins, iron, zinc.

▌PAWPAW, PINEAPPLE ▌AND MANGO

This juice has two of my other favourite island fruits and makes a deliciously sweet, fragrant juice. Pineapple makes the pawpaw and mango into a more liquid juice and, therefore, easier to drink. Together, these fruits make a potent antioxidant and protective juice – one which is also deeply cleansing and soothing for the digestive system.

1 pawpaw
1 mango
¼ pineapple

■ Peel all the skins and remove stones and seeds. Chop into juicer-sized chunks. This juice will naturally form coloured tiers of red, orange and yellow. Stir the mixture well and drink it immediately.
Rich in beta-carotene, bromelian, folic acid, vitamin C, calcium, phosphorus, flavonoids, magnesium and potassium.
Traces of B vitamins, iron, zinc and copper.

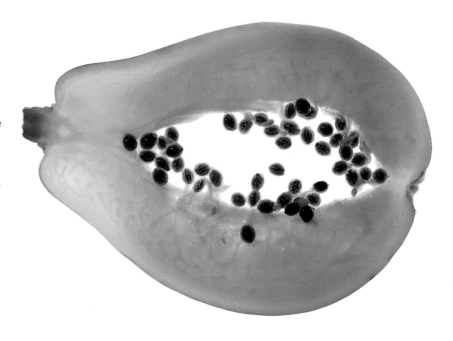

Grape

STRAIGHT GRAPE JUICE

This is a delicious, very sweet juice, full of energizing natural sugars, and easy to digest. Children love it. Its colour obviously depends on whether you use green or red grapes, but the more important consideration is ripeness. The riper the grapes, the sweeter and more plentiful the juice, and the richer it will be in nutrients. Grapes produce an antioxidant juice which, combined with its energizing properties, makes this a perfect drink for convalescents.

Large bunch of red or green grapes

■ Wash thoroughly, remove from the stalk and juice the grapes (including pips, if they have them). Drink the juice right after making it.
Rich in calcium, magnesium, phosphorus, flavonoids, potassium, vitamins C and E.
Traces of vitamins B1, B2, B3, copper, iron and zinc.

GRAPE AND PLUM

This is a beautiful red juice that tastes delicious. The addition of plums makes this an even more powerful antioxidant cocktail than the grapes alone. Plums are very soothing for the digestion, and contain lots of iron, so are good for the blood.

1 small bunch of red grapes
3–4 plums

■ Remove the grapes from the stalk, wash and stone the plums, and juice. Stir and drink this immediately.

Rich in beta-carotene, folic acid, calcium, magnesium, phosphorus, flavonoids, potassium, vitamins C and E. **Traces of** B1, B2, B3, iron, copper and zinc.

GRAPE, PINEAPPLE AND APRICOT

This sweetly delicious juice is deeply cleansing and packed with antioxidants for fighting infections. It is particularly cleansing for the digestive system and is both laxative and diuretic. Full of natural sugars, this is a very energizing and ideal breakfast drink.

1 small bunch of grapes
⅓ pineapple
2 apricots

■ Wash the grapes and apricots, removing the stones from the apricots but leaving the seeds in the grapes. Peel the pineapple. Cut it into chunks and juice. Drink the juice immediately.

Rich in beta-carotene, bromelian, folic acid, calcium, iron, magnesium, phosphorus, flavonoids, potassium and vitamins B3, B5, C and E. **Traces of** other B vitamins, copper and zinc.

Cherry

STRAIGHT CHERRY JUICE

Cherries are delicious – if a bit fiddly to prepare! For this reason, they tend to be added to other juices. But, if you can be bothered to stone them, the straight juice has a lovely sweet taste, as well as a delicious smell, too. Cherry juice is a natural antiseptic and has been known to alleviate problems such as arthritis and gout caused by excess uric acid. It is said to be a powerful cancer-fighter and to soothe headaches and migraines. This juice also has a softening and smoothing effect on the skin.

250g (½ lb) cherries

■ Wash, stone and juice the cherries. Drink immediately.
Rich in beta-carotene, folic acid, vitamin C, calcium, flavonoids, magnesium, phosphorus and potassium.

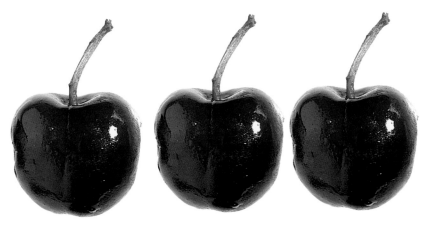

Traces of B vitamins, iron, zinc.

CHERRY AND NECTARINE

This is an absolutely delicious juice – really thick, with a strong, fruity flavour. Both antioxidant and cleansing, it is a good stress-buster and also good for allergy problems and headaches.

125g (¼ lb) cherries
3 nectarines

■ Wash, halve and stone the cherries and nectarines. Juice and drink immediately.
Rich in beta-carotene, folic acid, vitamin C, calcium, magnesium, flavonoids, phosphorus and potassium.
Traces of B vitamins, iron, zinc.

Kiwi

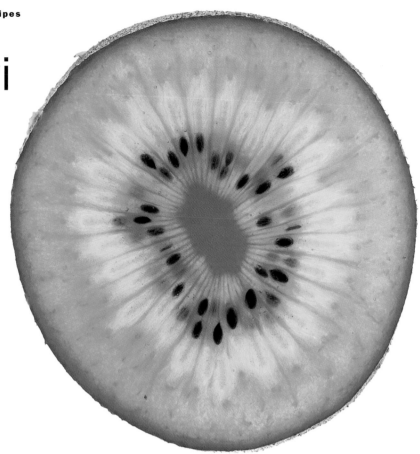

STRAIGHT KIWI JUICE

Kiwi fruit is packed with powerful nutrients; it is both energizing and deeply detoxifying. It boosts the immune system and improves digestion. Kiwi juice is great alone and as an addition to a number of juices. It is best to juice the kiwi with its skin on, from a nutritional point of view, but if you find that this makes the juice taste too bitter for you, then you can peel it.

3 kiwi fruits

■ Wash or peel and juice the fruit. Drink the juice immediately.
Rich in beta-carotene, vitamin C, magnesium, calcium, phosphorus, bioflavonoids, potassium.
Traces of B vitamins and iron.

KIWI AND PEAR

The combination of kiwi and pear produces a pale green, thick juice that is an excellent cleansing, immune system booster. Being a mild diuretic, the juice is useful for anyone with water retention problems. It tastes sweet with a tangy aftertaste.

1 kiwi fruit
1 large pear

■ Wash, cut into juicer-sized pieces, juice and drink immediately.
Rich in beta-carotene, folic acid, vitamin C, calcium, pectin, magnesium, bioflavonoids, phos-phorus and potassium.
Traces of B vitamins, iron, copper, manganese and zinc.

KIWI COCKTAIL

A cleansing and energizing thick, green juice; it is beneficial for the skin – ideal as a wrinkle remover.

3 kiwi fruits
Small bunch of grapes
1 apple
1 banana

■ Wash the kiwi fruit, apple and grapes (removing them from their stalks). Cut the apple and kiwi fruits to fit the juicer. Peel the banana and juice it first, followed by the kiwi fruit, grapes and the apple. Stir and drink immediately.
Rich in beta-carotene, folic acid, pectin, calcium, magnesium, phosphorus, potassium and vitamins C and E.
Traces of B vitamins, iron and zinc.

Mango

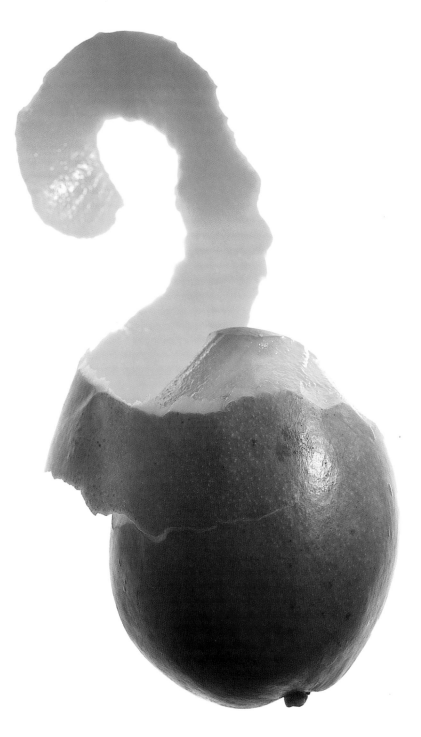

STRAIGHT MANGO JUICE

Like pawpaw juice, this is one that you really need a spoon to drink, it's so thick and rich. Mango juice is highly antioxidant and so protective of your health generally, and is said to counter-act some cancers. In particular, it benefits the kidneys and cleanses the blood. Because it's so thick it is normally mixed with other juices, but to make a quick but heavenly drink, use:

2–3 mangoes

■ Peel the mangoes, remove their stones and juice the fruit. Stir and drink immediately.
Rich in beta-carotene, vitamin C, calcium, magnesium and potassium.
Traces of B vitamins, iron, copper and zinc.

MANGO COCKTAIL

This thick, deliciously sweet juice comes out as a yellow-green colour. It's packed full of antioxidants and so is a great immune system booster and will give you beautiful skin. Make sure that all of the ingredients you use – particulary the mango itself – are ripe.

1 mango
1 banana
1 kiwi fruit
2 apples

■ Peel the mango and remove the stone. Peel the banana, scrub the kiwi (or peel, if you prefer) and apples. Juice, then stir as you drink as this juice tends to separate.

Rich in beta-carotene, folic acid, pectin, calcium, magnesium, phosphorus, potassium, bioflavonoids, vitamins B3, C, E.
Traces of B vitamins, iron, manganese, copper and zinc.

Melon

STRAIGHT MELON JUICE

There are numerous varieties of melon but all are delicious. Melon has a very high water content and so goes through the body at great speed, cleansing and rehydrating it while, at the same time, removing bloating and puffiness.

1 small melon

■ Peel and cut the melon into juicer-sized pieces. Juice, with pips. Drink immediately.
Rich in beta-carotene, folic acid, vitamin C, calcium, chlorine, magnesium, phosphorus and potassium.
Traces of B vitamins, iron, zinc, vitamin E and copper.

MELON AND GRAPE

This is a sweet, fragrant juice, whose quality depends on the type of melon you use. The Ogen and Galia varieties will yield the best juice. Melon juice is cleansing and restorative.

½ melon
Small bunch of grapes

■ Remove the peel from the melon with a knife and cut into slices that will fit into the juicer. You can juice the seeds, too, if you wish. Pick the grapes from the stalk and wash them. Drink this immediately after juicing.
Rich in beta-carotene, folic acid, calcium, magnesium, phosphorus, potassium and vitamins C and E.
Traces of B vitamins, iron, zinc and copper.

MELON AND PLUM

Another very sweet juice (you can leave out the banana if you want). It is energizing and has plenty of iron, making it useful for women during menstruation.

¼ sweet melon
1 plum
1 kiwi fruit
1 banana

■ Remove the peel from the melon with a knife and cut it into slices, keeping or omitting the seeds as you prefer. Wash the plum, cut it in half and remove the stone. Peel the banana. Scrub the kiwi fruit, then cut it in half. I prefer to leave the skin on the kiwi fruit, but, if you find that you don't like the slightly peppery after-taste that it gives the drink, you can peel it. Drink the juice immediately.
Rich in beta-carotene, folic acid, calcium, magnesium, phosphorus, potassium and vitamins C and E.
Traces of B vitamins, copper, iron and zinc.

MELON AND STRAWBERRY

This juice is antiviral, a powerful antioxidant, a cancer-fighter and is said to be beneficial for arthritis. A pale fondant pink with a creamy texture, it's sweetly delicious, especially if you use a Galia or Ogen melon.

¼ melon
1 punnet of strawberries

■ Wash the strawberries, peel and chop the melon. Juice, including the melon seeds, and drink immediately.
Rich in beta-carotene, folic acid, biotin, calcium, chlorine, magnesium, phosphorus, potassium and vitamins E, C and K.
Traces of B vitamins, iron, copper and zinc.

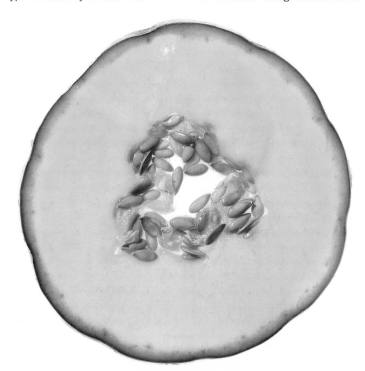

Peach

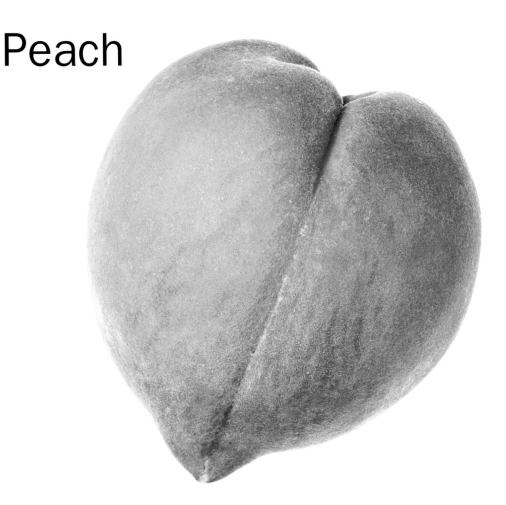

STRAIGHT PEACH JUICE

Peaches make a thick, sweet, delicious juice – but it is important always to choose ripe ones. They have a deeply cleansing effect, notably on the kidneys and bladder, and are energizing, slightly diuretic and laxative, but quite soothing to the digestive system at the same time. This makes them a good way to boost the body for overall detoxification purposes. The ingredients for a small, rich juice are simply:

3 peaches

■ Wash, remove the stones and juice the fruit. Drink this immediately.
Rich in beta-carotene, folic acid, calcium, magnesium, phosphorus, potassium and vitamins B3 and C.
Traces of B vitamins, copper, iron and zinc.

PEACH AND PERSIMMON

This is a nectar of a juice – just make sure you use ripe fruit. Persimmons have a high beta-carotene and vitamin C content, as do peaches, and together they make a highly protective, immune system boosting juice which is thick, bright orange and very sweet.

1 peach
1 persimmon

■ Wash the fruit thoroughly and remove the stone from the peach. Juice, stir and drink immediately.
Rich in beta-carotene, folic acid, calcium, magnesium, phosphorus, potassium and vitamins B3 and C.
Traces of B vitamins, copper, iron and zinc.

Orange

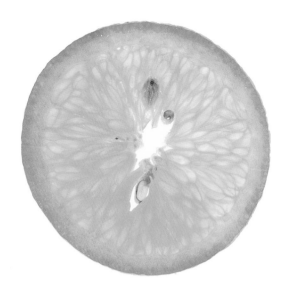

STRAIGHT ORANGE JUICE

The most popular of all juices, it is an excellent antioxidant and toner. Orange juice stimulates the heart, circulation and the digestive system, and counteracts constipation. However, too much of this acidic juice can upset the acid-alkaline ratio of the body. It is better, therefore, to drink it every other day at most, with other, more alkaline, juices in-between.

3 oranges

■ If you have a citrus juicer, just cut the oranges in half and juice. If you are using a regular juicer, you must peel them, removing most of the pith. Drink immediately.
Rich in beta-carotene, vitamins B1, B6 and C, folic acid, cal-cium, magnesium, iron, phosphorus and potassium.
Traces of other B vitamins, vitamin E and zinc.

ORANGE AND CARROT

Not surprisingly, this is a very orange juice. It has great antioxidant powers, the carrots balancing the acidity of the orange. Profoundly cleansing and energizing, this juice stimulates the body to fight off infection and increase cell renewal.

2 oranges
3 carrots

■ Peel the oranges and scrub the carrots. Drink this immediately after juicing them. If you find this too sweet, add a few leaves of mint.

Rich in beta-carotene, vitamins B1, B6 and C, folic acid, iron, calcium, magnesium and potassium.
Traces of other B vitamins, vitamin E and zinc.

ORANGE BREAKFAST

This perfect antioxidant, cleansing, sweet, bright orange wake-up juice gives you a burst of instant energy.

1 slice of pineapple
1 nectarine
2 oranges

■ Peel the oranges and pineapple and cut into slices. Wash the nectarine and remove the stone. Juice the orange last. Stir and drink immediately after juicing.
Rich in beta-carotene, bromelian, folic acid, calcium, magnesium, iron, phosphorus, potassium, vitamins B6 and C.
Traces of other B vitamins, vitamin E and zinc.

ORANGE AND BANANA

Another good early morning drink, especially since the banana is so energizing and takes away the acidity of the oranges. The antiseptic qualities of the orange combine with the antibiotic properties of the banana for a really protective, health-giving juice.

4 oranges
1 banana

■ Peel and remove the pith from the oranges and the banana. Juice the banana first, then the oranges. Stir before drinking this.
Rich in beta-carotene, iron, folic acid, calcium, magnesium, phosphorus, potassium and vitamins B1, B6, K and C.
Traces of other B vitamins, vitamin E and zinc.

ORANGE AND GRAPEFRUIT

High in vitamin C, this is an excellent immune system booster, although it's only for those who don't insist on a super-sweet juice, as it has a sharp kick!

1 grapefruit
2 oranges

■ Peel the fruit, remove the pith. Cut into chunks, juice and drink immediately.
Rich in beta-carotene, folic acid, calcium, magnesium, phosphorus, iron, potassium and vitamins B1, B6 and C.
Traces of E and B vitamins, manganese, copper and zinc.

Mandarin

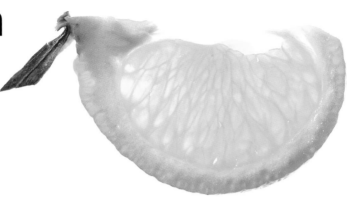

STRAIGHT MANDARIN JUICE

Mandarin juice is sweeter than orange, so children usually prefer it. With most of the same nutrients as orange juice, it is a good all-round health protector and energizer. The added ingredient of ginger stimulates the circulation and is generally warming, so it is a good juice for starting a winter's day.

6 mandarins
½ inch ginger root

■ Peel the mandarins. Scrub the ginger with an abrasive surface. Juice and drink this immediately.
Rich in beta-carotene, folic acid, calcium, magnesium, phosphorus, potassium and vitamins B6 and C.
Traces of other B vitamins, vitamin E and zinc.

Nectarine

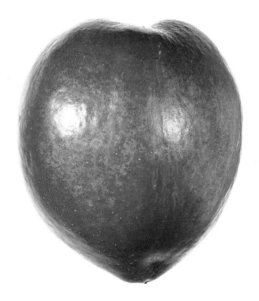

STRAIGHT NECTARINE JUICE

Like the peach, the nectarine produces only a small amount of thick, rich sweet juice. For this reason, nectarines are usually juiced with fruits that have a higher water content, but it does make a deliciously fragrant juice all by itself as well. The taste and texture is similar to peach and the juice has similar properties, being both a detoxifier and booster to the immune system. The ingredients for this juice are very simple:

4 nectarines

■ Wash the fruit thoroughly under running water, remove the stones, juice and drink immediately.
Rich in beta-carotene, folic acid, vitamin C, calcium, magnesium, phosphorus and potassium.
Traces of B vitamins, iron and zinc.

NECTARINE AND PINEAPPLE

Nectarines' rich, sweet taste combines with the pineapple, making a rich, creamy orange-yellow nectar. Granadilla gives this cleansing, energizing juice an unusual taste and lessens sweetness.

2 nectarines
¼ large pineapple
1 granadilla or passion fruit

■ Wash the nectarines and remove the stones. Peel the pineapple and cut it into chunks that will fit comfortably in your juicer. Scoop out the granadilla. Juice, stir and drink immediately.
Rich in beta-carotene, bromelian, folic acid, vitamin C, calcium, magnesium, phosphorus and potassium.
Traces of B vitamins, iron and zinc.

Watermelon

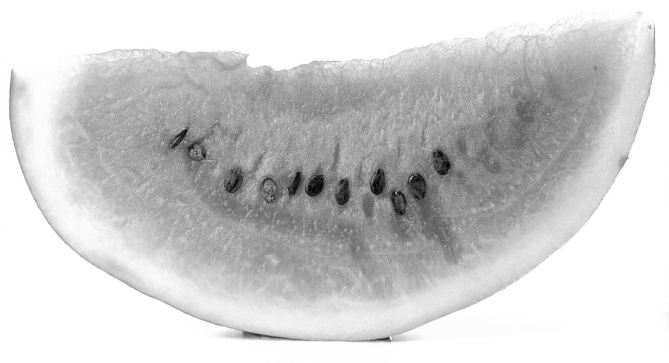

STRAIGHT WATERMELON JUICE

This pretty, light, sweet pink juice can be quite a mess in the making! Because watermelon has such a high water content, it tends to overflow out of the juicer and to spray seeds as you feed it into the machine. This drink is very useful for counter-acting water retention and bloat-ing, and has a calming effect on the mind and the emotions.

⅛ watermelon

■ Remove the rind but keep the seeds. Cut into chunks. Juice and drink immediately.
Rich in beta-carotene, vitamins C and B5, folic acid, calcium, magnesium, phosphorus and potassium.
Traces of B vitamins, iron and zinc.

WATERMELON AND BLACKBERRIES

The blackberries make this a powerfully cleansing antioxidant. It's a dark red, somewhat sweet, thin juice.

⅛ watermelon
1 punnet of blackberries

■ Wash the blackberries thoroughly under running water and put through the juicer. Remove the rind from the watermelon and juice the melon. It is important to remember to include its seeds. Stir well and drink this juice immediately.
Rich in beta-carotene, vitamins C, E and B5, folic acid, sodium, calcium, magnesium, phos-phorus and potassium.
Traces of B vitamins, copper, iron and zinc.

WATERMELON AND CHERRIES

A delicious, dark red, sweet juice which is very good for the skin and for reducing stress.

⅛ watermelon
125g (¼lb) cherries

■ Wash the cherries thoroughly under running water and then remove their stones. Remove the rind from the watermelon and chop the flesh into chunks that will fit in the juicer. Remember not to discard the seeds – they are an important ingredient. Juice and drink immediately.
Rich in beta-carotene, vitamins C and B5 folic acid, calcium, magnesium, phosphorus and potassium.
Traces of B vitamins, iron and zinc.

Banana

Bananas, to be strictly truthful, don't juice; they pulp. They produce a thick, almost solid, substance that sinks to the bottom of all mixes and needs to be stirred in thoroughly. However, the delicious sweetness and fragrance of banana "juice" is such that it's used in lots of recipes to overcome more tart fruits. It lowers cholesterol, is a super-energizer and a natural antibiotic, and I would recommend putting banana in any mix that isn't sweet already. It is vital, though, always to use ripe bananas – the ones, in fact, that are turning brown and speckled, and that you'd rather not eat.

BANANA AND MELON

This is a super-sweet, cleansing and energizing juice that is particularly good as a breakfast drink for children. For the best results, always choose a ripe melon and banana.

2 bananas
½ melon
1 apple

■ Wash the apple and peel the bananas and melon. Put through the juicer one banana, followed by some melon, followed by the second banana and then the remaining ingredients. Bananas yield very little liquid, but this way you get the most from them. Stir well.

Rich in beta-carotene, folic acid, calcium, magnesium, phosphorus, potassium and vitamins C and K.
Traces of other B vitamins, iron and zinc.

BANANA AND KIWI

The kiwi fruits make this a thick, green juice. It is very sweet and creamy, energizing, stimulating to the digestive system, and a powerful antioxidant as well.

2 bananas
2 kiwi fruits
1 apple

■ Peel the bananas and juice them first. Wash and cut the kiwi fruits and apple to fit the juicer. Juice, stir and drink immediately.

Rich in beta-carotene, folic acid, calcium, magnesium, phosphorus, potassium and vitamins C and E.
Traces of other B vitamins, zinc and iron.

BANANA AND CRANBERRY

The sweetness of the banana balances the tartness of the cranberry well. It also is a very beneficial juice. Cranberries cleanse the kidneys, bladder and urinary tract, and combat urinary infections efficiently; they also are said to contain cancer-fighting chemicals. Bananas and pineapples are deep cleansers. Rather surprisingly, as bananas are always thought of as energizing, they can also help you sleep, so this is a good night-time drink especially if you suffer from kidney or urinary problems.

½ punnet of cranberries
One thick slice of pineapple
2 bananas

■ Wash thoroughly and remove the stalks from all the cranberries. Remove the peel from the pineapple and bananas and cut into juicer-sized chunks. Juice, stir and drink this immediately.

Rich in beta-carotene, folic acid, bromelian, calcium, magnesium, phosphorus, potassium and vitamins C and E.
Traces of other B vitamins, zinc and iron.

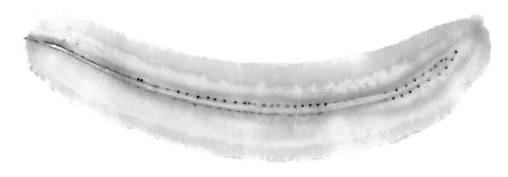

Pineapple

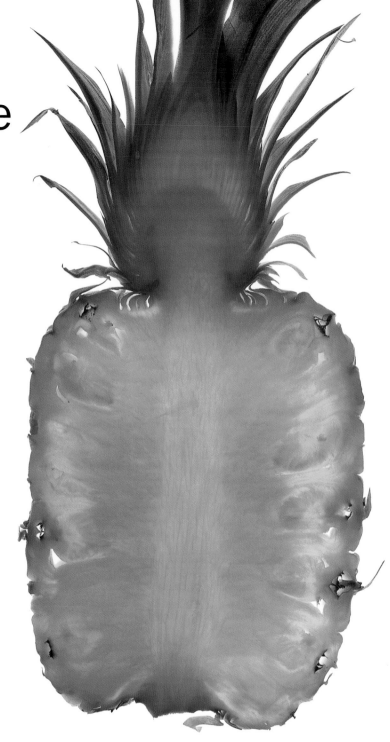

STRAIGHT PINEAPPLE JUICE

Like orange, pineapple juice is widely available ready-made in supermarkets. Freshly made, however, it's a very different drink – sweet and thick with a divine fragrance. It has plenty of natural sugars, it is always energizing, stimulates the body to heal and renew itself on a cellular level, and promotes good digestion. Always buy a ripe pineapple. Discard the leaves and skin, and juice the core.

½ pineapple

■ Peel the tough outer skin of the pineapple and discard it together with the leaves. Chop into chunks suitable for the size of your juicer, juice and drink immediately.
Rich in beta-carotene, folic acid, vitamin C, bromelian, calcium, magnesium, phosphorus and potassium.
Traces of B vitamins, iron and zinc.

PINEAPPLE, BANANA AND APPLE

This is a lovely, pale yellow, cream-textured juice that is very sweet and thick. Both banana and pineapple are deeply energizing, so this is a good breakfast juice. It is very cleansing, stimulates the digestive system and also lowers cholesterol.

1 thick slice of pineapple
1 banana
1 apple

■ Remove the pineapple skin, then slice. Wash the apple and peel the banana, juicing the banana first and the apple last. Stir and drink immediately. You may have to stir the juice many times as the banana will sink.
Rich in beta-carotene, folic acid, pectin, bromelian, calcium, magnesium, phosphorus, potassium and vitamins B6, C and K.
Traces of B vitamins, iron and zinc.

Plum

STRAIGHT PLUM JUICE

This delicious, fragrant juice with a distinctive golden colour is highly antioxidant. Along with its iron content, this makes it very useful for protecting overall health, avoiding anaemia, generally strengthening the blood, and improving digestion. All you need is:

5–6 plums

■ Wash the plums, then cut them in half and remove their stones. Drink this juice immediately after juicing.
Rich in beta-carotene, folic acid, calcium, magnesium, phosphorus, potassium and vitamins C and E.
Traces of B vitamins and iron.

PLUM AND PINEAPPLE

This very cleansing, healing juice, bursting with vitamin C, also happens to taste delicious. Leave the skin on the kiwi fruit for a slightly peppery aftertaste, or remove it if you prefer just a plain sweet drink. This drink acts as a general antioxidant and can normalize the digestive system if it has been upset.

2 plums
1 thick slice of pineapple
1 kiwi fruit

■ Remove the skin from the pineapple, then cut the fruit into slices. Wash the plums and kiwi fruit (peel them if you do not want a peppery taste) and remove the plum stones. Juice, stir, and to reap its full benefit, drink immediately.

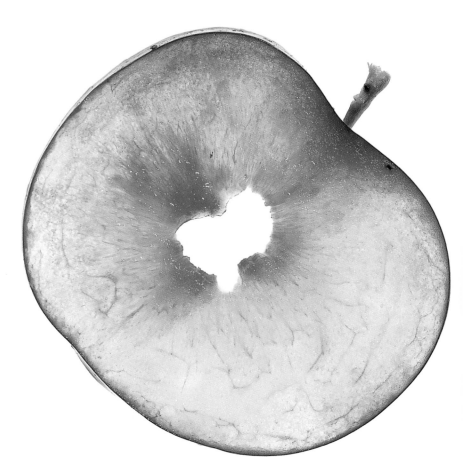

Rich in beta-carotene, folic acid, bromelian, calcium, magnesium, phosphorus, potassium, vitamins C and E.
Traces of B vitamins and iron.

PLUM, APPLE AND FIG

It's almost a pudding, this delicious sweet purple juice is so thick and rich. This is a very effective juice for overcoming constipation and helps to balance the digestive system. Make sure, however, that the figs are ripe.

2 plums
1 apple
2–3 figs

■ Scoop the flesh of the figs out from its peel and then juice them first, followed by the washed, stoned plums and seeded apple. Stir well and drink the juice as soon as you have made it.
Rich in beta-carotene, folic acid, pectin, calcium, iron, magnesium, phosphorus, potassium and vitamins C and E.
Traces of B vitamins, zinc and copper.

Raspberry

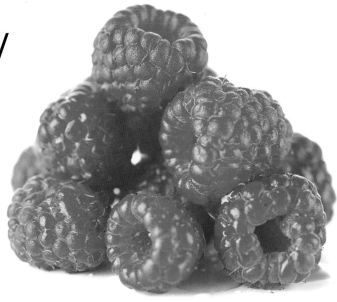

▌STRAIGHT RASPBERRY JUICE

This is a delicious juice, very fragrant and not too sweet, but, because it's very thick, it tends to be used in mixes. Although you can drink it straight, you don't get much juice from raspberries, so buy them when they're in season and cheapest. They will also be at their ripest then, and so at their best nutritionally. Packed with antioxidants, they promote all-round health, but are principally known for their benefits to women's health, and can help with period pain.

2 punnets of raspberries

■ Wash, juice, drink.
Rich in beta-carotene, biotin, chlorine, calcium, iron, magnesium, phosphorus, potassium and vitamin C.
Traces of other B vitamins, vitamin E and copper.

▌RASPBERRY AND QUINCE

This combination is particularly beneficial for relieving indigestion. However, quince does not yield much juice, and it needs to be very ripe for any to be squeezed out at all. The addition of quince reinforces the antioxidant properties of raspberries.

1 punnet of raspberries
1 quince

■ Wash and cut the quince into small pieces. Juice all the fruit and drink immediately.
Rich in beta-carotene, biotin, chlorine, calcium, iron, magnesium, phosphorus, potassium and vitamin C.
Traces of other B vitamins, vitamin E and copper.

▌RASPBERRY AND APPLE

This is a bright pink, fruity juice, but not too sweet because it has a slight tang from the raspberries. To make it sweeter, add an extra banana. A very cleansing juice, it is good for a detoxification fast, and can combat cold symptoms. If you have a cold, take this juice last thing at night and the banana's natural tryptophan will help you to sleep.

1 punnet of raspberries
3 apples
1 banana

■ Wash the raspberries and apples thoroughly under running water, then cut the apples into chunks. Peel the banana and juice it first, then the raspberries, and finally the apples. Mix well and drink the juice immediately.
Rich in beta-carotene, biotin, chlorine, pectin, folic acid, calcium, iron, magnesium, phosphorus, potassium and vitamin C.
Traces of other B vitamins, vitamin E, copper and zinc.

▌RASPBERRY AND MELON

This thick, sweet, pink juice is instantly energizing and cleansing for the body. It is very good as a diuretic and mild laxative. Raspberries can make a somewhat bitter drink, but a sweet melon and a banana make this delicious.

1 punnet of raspberries
¼ sweet melon
1 banana

■ Wash the raspberries, peel the banana and juice them both, banana first. Remove the rind from the melon, but remember to juice the fruit with its seeds. Stir and drink immediately.
Rich in beta-carotene, biotin, chlorine, folic acid, calcium, iron, magnesium, phosphorus, potassium and vitamin C.
Traces of other B vitamins and vitamin E, copper and zinc.

Strawberry

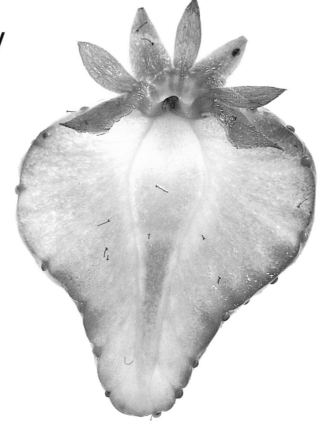

STRAIGHT STRAWBERRY JUICE

It's an amazing piece of luck that something so delicious can also be so good for you! Strawberries have great antioxidant powers, and are also said to fight off cancers, bacteria and viruses. They are beneficial for arthritis and even have an in-built painkiller! Always buy in season, but be aware that they don't produce much juice.

2 punnets of strawberries

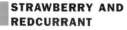 Wash, juice, drink.
Rich in beta-carotene, folic acid, biotin, calcium, magnesium, phosphorus, chlorine, potassium, vitamins C and E.
Traces of B vitamins, iron, zinc.

STRAWBERRY AND REDCURRANT

The sweetness of strawberries balances well with redcurrants' tartness in this infection-fighting juice. It is particularly beneficial in cases of fever.

1 punnet of strawberries
1 punnet of redcurrants

■ Wash the berries thoroughly under running water and remove all stalks. Juice the fruit and drink immediately.
Rich in beta-carotene, folic acid, biotin, calcium, magnesium, phosphorus, chlorine, potas-sium, vitamins C and E.
Traces of B vitamins, iron, zinc.

BERRIES AND CHERRIES

This is a deliciously sweet juice which, besides its far-reaching health benefits, also has anti-ageing properties by helping to soften lines and wrinkles on the skin. For the best results, make sure that the fruit you use is ripe; the general rule is that if it's not ready for eating, then it's not ready for juicing either.

½ punnet of strawberries
½ punnet of raspberries
125g (¼lb) cherries
1 peach

■ Wash all the fruit thoroughly in warm water and remove the stones from the peach and cherries. Juice in any order, stir and serve.
Rich in beta-carotene, folic acid, calcium, magnesium, chlorine, biotin, phosphorus, potassium, and vitamins B3, E and C.
Traces of copper, manganese, zinc and vitamins B1, B2, B5 and B6.

BERRIES AND WATERMELON

This delicious, sweet, light-tasting, thick juice is an ideal cooling drink for a hot summer's day. An excellent all-round health juice, it is also very effective for curing water retention and for combating constipation. Furthermore, it is a valuable rehydrating juice.

1 punnet of strawberries
1 punnet of redcurrants
¼ watermelon

■ Wash the strawberries and redcurrants. Remove the rind from the watermelon. Juice all fruits (including watermelon seeds), then drink this immediately.
Rich in beta-carotene, folic acid, biotin, calcium, magnesium, phosphorus, potassium, chlorine and vitamins B5, C and E.
Traces of B vitamins, iron, zinc.

Carrot

STRAIGHT CARROT JUICE

Carrot juice is superbly good for you. It is extremely energizing, a potent antioxidant, is said to protect against infection and certain cancers, and dissolves ulcers. As a detoxifier, it cleanses the main organs of detoxification – the liver and kidneys – and the entire digestive tract. It is also an aid for building up red blood corpuscles and is excellent for the skin. However, if you drink too much of it, you can start to turn orange from the pigment in the carrots! So, for this and other reasons, I mix it with other fruit or vegetables which reinforce its health-giving powers but tone down its taste slightly, which can be a bit too sweet and overwhelming. (To avoid this, sprinkle some iron-rich spirulina into it.)

5 carrots

■ Scrub and juice the carrots, leaving on their top leaves if they are organic. Drink immediately.
Rich in beta-carotene, folic acid, vitamin C, magnesium, calcium, and potassium.
Traces of B vitamins, iron and zinc.

CARROT AND APPLE

One of the few occasions when you can mix fruit with a vegetable, carrot and apple juice is not only delicious, but one of

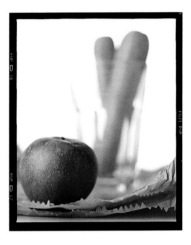

the best detoxifiers and immune system boosters you will ever find. This juice is also good as a beauty juice, since it is very good for your skin! Red apples will give it a sweet flavour, but carrots are very sweet when juiced, so you may prefer to use a tarter apple, for example, a Granny Smith.

4 carrots
2 large apples

■ Scrub the carrots and wash the apples, leaving tops on organic carrots. Juice the carrots first, and then the apples. Stir and drink immediately.
Rich in beta-carotene, folic acid, vitamin C, calcium, pectin, magnesium, potassium and phosphorus.
Traces of vitamins B1, B2, B3, B6, E, copper, iron and zinc.

CARROT AND KIWI

This juice is highly antioxidant, protective, and diuretic. It is also deeply cleansing.

3 carrots
2 apples
2 kiwi fruits

■ Wash the carrots and apples thoroughly under running water. Cut them into juicer-sized pieces. If you like the peppery taste of kiwi fruit skin, just scrub, cut in half and juice the fruit. If not, peel it. Stir and drink the juice immediately.
Rich in beta-carotene, vitamin C, folic acid, calcium, pectin, magnesium, potassium and phosphorus.
Traces of B vitamins, vitamin E, iron and zinc.

HERBY CARROT

The herbs used in this drink add extra nutrients to the carrot juice, making it a great health booster. Parsley is a particularly powerful antioxidant which adds a stronger, fresher flavour to the sweetness of the carrots and is also an excellent diuretic that helps to relieve water retention.

6 carrots
One handful each of mint and parsley

■ Wash the carrots and herbs, then juice them, including all organic leaves. Stir and drink immediately.
Rich in beta-carotene, vitamin C, calcium, magnesium, potas-sium and folic acid.
Traces of B vitamins, iron and zinc.

Beetroot

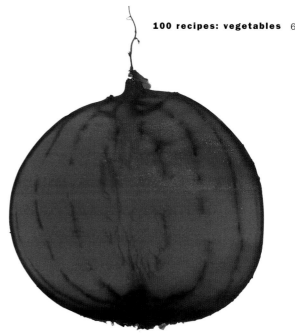

STRAIGHT BEETROOT JUICE

One of the greatest cleansers and immune system boosters, beetroot juice works powerfully against kidney stones, gall bladder and liver problems, and strengthens the blood, which means that it is good for problems like anaemia. It is also a great energizer, as it is full of natural sugars, but, because so many people don't like to eat beetroot, it is far less widely drunk than it should be. In fact, even people who don't like to eat this vegetable often find its juice quite palatable. It is sweet and at the same time earthy-tasting. Its bright purple colour can amaze you the first time you see it, and, even when mixed with other juices, beetroot has a tendency to turn urine a pretty shade of pink!

3 medium beetroots

■ Scrub, but don't peel or remove the leaves and roots (if organic). Juice and drink immediately.

BEETROOT AND CUCUMBER

This juice retains its astonishing beetroot colour. This extremely valuable antioxidant juice also acts as a diuretic due to the addition of cucumber. It is said to lower blood pressure, too, and is a general aid for digestion.

2 beetroots
½ cucumber
2 celery stalks, including leaves
Half a small bunch of watercress

■ Wash all the vegetables, giving the beetroot a good scrub. Don't peel anything and keep all the organic leaves, tops and stalks. Put the watercress into the juicer first, followed by the beetroot, celery and cucumber. If the taste of the watercress seems very strong, or too bitter, use the other half of the cucumber to dilute it. Stir and drink immediately.
Rich in beta-carotene, folic acid, vitamins C and B6, calcium, silica and potassium.
Traces of vitamins B1, B2, B3, B5, iron and zinc.

BEETROOT AND CARROT

This is a purple-red, sweet, earthy juice that is great for the immune system and very high in vitamins and minerals.

2 beetroots
2 carrots
Handful of parsley

■ Scrub the beetroots and carrots, leaving on organic leaves for juicing. Wash the parsley. Juice and drink immediately.

Rich in beta-carotene, folic acid, vitamins B6 and C, calcium, magnesium, iron and potassium.
Traces of other B vitamins, iron and zinc.

BEETROOT AND SPINACH

Because it is so sweet, beetroot takes the bitterness out of spinach, which otherwise can be difficult as a juice. The celery adds a tangy, peppery flavour.

2 beetroots
Large handful of spinach
2 sticks of celery

■ Scrub the beetroot and celery, leaving on organic leaves. Wash the spinach thoroughly. Juice each alternately, as spinach is very fibrous and will block many smaller juicers if you put through too much at one time. Stir to mix and drink immediately.
Rich in beta-carotene, folic acid, B3, B6, vitamin C, calcium, iron, potassium.
Traces of other B vitamins, vitamin E, iron and zinc.

Broccoli

Broccoli can easily be regarded as a wonder juice, it has so many functions. It is a powerful antioxidant and warrior against cancer, a natural antibiotic, and a deep cleanser, particularly for the liver, the body's most important organ of detoxification. Because it is so deeply cleansing, it has a rejuvenating effect on the skin, too. It is too bitter to drink on its own, so it should always be mixed with something sweeter – carrots or beetroot are ideal and reinforce its health-giving properties with their own. You can use either green or purple-sprouting broccoli to make the following juices.

BROCCOLI AND BEETROOT

This is a potent health juice, working as an antioxidant, cancer fighter and deep cleanser.

It is particularly good for cleaning toxins from the liver and strengthens the blood. The addition of fennel makes this juice useful for losing weight, while lettuce provides it with diuretic qualities.

6 large lettuce leaves
1 head of broccoli
Handful of chard (or spring greens)
1 small beetroot
½ bulb of fennel

■ Wash all of the ingredients and chop everything into juicer-sized pieces, leaving on organic leaves. Juice, stir and drink immediately.
Rich in beta-carotene, folic acid, calcium, iron, sodium, magnesium, phosphorus, potassium and vitamins B3, B5, B6 and C.
Traces of other B vitamins, copper and zinc.

BROCCOLI, CARROT AND PEPPER

The sweetness of the carrot and pepper balances the bitterness of the broccoli, making this a pleasant-tasting juice. It is a good general detoxification juice and has powerful health-protecting qualities. It is a real skin beautifier and eye brightener as well.

1 large head of broccoli
2 large carrots
1 red pepper

■ Wash the vegetables and remove the stalk and seeds from the pepper. Chop into juicer-sized pieces, juice, stir and drink immediately.
Rich in beta-carotene, folic acid, vitamin C, calcium, iron, magnesium, sodium and potassium.
Traces of B vitamins, vitamin E and zinc.

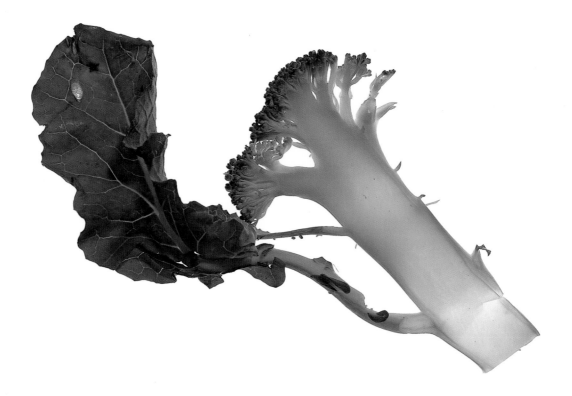

Cabbage

Cabbage juice has too strong a taste to drink on its own; you always need to mix it with sweeter juices. Different types of cabbage will produce different types of juice and benefits. Green cabbage has the strongest, most bitter taste, while red is peppery and white is the sweetest. All of the cabbage family are said to have powerful antioxidant, cancer-protecting properties and help build up immunity to disease. They are also great cleansers and good for the digestive tract and the skin, in particular.

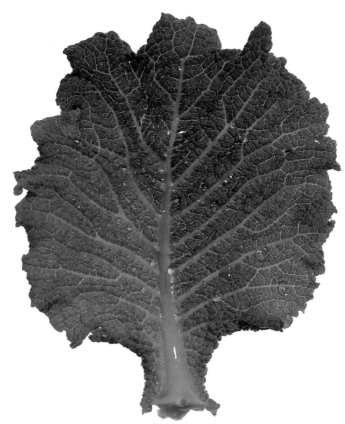

■ CABBAGE AND SWEET POTATO

This is a light, frothy juice with an equally light, pleasant taste. It tends to separate, so keep stirring as you drink it.

½ small cabbage
1 sweet potato
2 tomatoes

■ Wash the cabbage leaves and tomatoes and give the sweet potato a good scrub, removing any damaged areas. The cabbage will be the toughest to juice, so intersperse it with the sweet potato and tomatoes. Stir and drink it immediately.
Rich in beta-carotene, folic acid, chlorine, biotin, calcium, magnesium, phosphorus, potassium, sodium and vitamins C and E.
Traces of B vitamins, sulphur, iron and zinc.

■ CABBAGE AND CELERY

A thin, light juice with a pleasant, slightly peppery aftertaste from the celery, it is a good general detoxifier, particularly for the digestive tract. This is another important antioxidant, cancer-fighting juice.

½ small cabbage
2 sticks of celery
2 tomatoes

■ Wash the vegetables thoroughly under running water, making sure you keep the organic leaves on the celery. Again, the cabbage is the toughest to juice, so put the celery and tomatoes through your juicer between batches of cabbage to prevent it blocking up. Stir and drink this juice immediately.
Rich in beta-carotene, folic acid, biotin, calcium, magnesium, manganese, potassium, sodium, chlorine and vitamins C and E.
Traces of B vitamins, sulphur, iron and zinc.

■ CABBAGE, QUINCE AND CARROT

This is a cleansing, antioxidant juice which is very soothing to the digestive system and particularly useful for combating gas. It is beneficial, also, as a stimulant to the body, and the parsley acts as a breath freshener. The quince will yield very little juice; try to find one as ripe as possible.

1 quince
Large handful of parsley
½ cabbage
2 carrots

■ Wash the ingredients thoroughly, juice them and drink immediately.
Rich in beta-carotene, folic acid, calcium, magnesium, potassium, sodium and vitamins C and E.
Traces of other B vitamins, iron and zinc.

Tomato

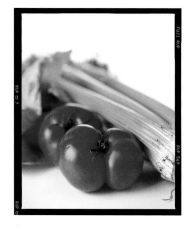

STRAIGHT TOMATO JUICE

Tomato is a well-known juice, but, freshly made, bears little resemblance to what you find in supermarkets. It has a sweet, fresh taste and a pink colour. It is also a rehydrating juice and a powerful antioxidant immune system booster.

6 tomatoes

■ Wash the tomatoes, remove their stalks, juice and drink.
Rich in beta-carotene, folic acid, vitamin C, biotin, calcium, magnesium, chlorine, potassium, sodium and vitamin E.

Traces of B vitamins, iron and zinc.

TOMATO AND CELERY

This is the innocent version of a Bloody Mary! Celery contains natural sodium, which gives this juice its delicious piquancy, and helps to lower blood pressure. It is a fresh, light juice, but the tomatoes and celery separate so keep mixing it as you drink.

6 large tomatoes
2 sticks of celery

■ Wash the ingredients, leaving any leaves on the celery. Juice the celery, then the tomatoes.
Rich in beta-carotene, folic acid, vitamin C, calcium, magnesium, chlorine, biotin, sodium, potassium, manganese and vitamin E.
Traces of vitamins B1, B2, B3, B5, B6, E, iron and zinc.

Watercress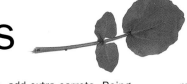

Watercress makes one of the most healing and protective juices around, and contains some of the highest levels of vitamins and minerals. An excellent detoxifier and blood purifier, it is also incredibly strong in terms of taste, so use it with great care! It does not produce a great quantity of juice, but what it does make has an eye-watering effect, so it should never form more than one-sixth of any combination. Rocket and dandelion can be substituted for watercress in order to create a slightly different flavour.

WATERCRESS AND CARROT

This juice packs quite a punch – even with the carrots to make it milder. If it's still too strong for you, add extra carrots. Being a lover of peppery tastes, I actually find it quite palatable – but sip, don't gulp it. Don't let its thin consistency and murky green colour repel you. It is particularly good for colds or throat infections (you can feel the burn on the way down!) or as a general pick-me-up.

½ bunch of watercress
1 large turnip
2 carrots

■ Wash all of the vegetables, then juice them, alternating between them in order to push the fibrous watercress through your juicer. If it is very frothy or you don't like the look of the froth, skim it off, stir and drink.
Rich in beta-carotene, vitamins C and E, calcium, sodium, iron, magnesium, phosphorus, folic acid and potassium.
Traces of B vitamins, zinc and copper.

WATERCRESS AND APPLE

This is a great detoxifier. It cleanses the blood, lowers cholesterol, breaks up stones in the kidney and bladder, and acts as a diuretic and laxative.

½ bunch watercress
3 sweet apples

■ Wash, juice, drink.
Rich in beta-carotene, pectin, folic acid, sodium, iron, calcium, magnesium, phosphorus, potassium, vitamins C and E.
Traces of B vitamins, zinc and copper.

Celery

Celery juice alone is rather strong and peppery, so always mix it with something a little sweeter, such as carrot or tomato. It is deeply cleansing, has a beneficial effect upon the nervous and blood systems, and promotes kidney function. It also has a soothing quality, so is very good in times of stress.

CELERY, CABBAGE AND CARROT

This juice contains some powerful nutrients, and is antioxidant and cleansing. It is a good juice for times when you are convalescing or suffering from an infection, particularly of the throat.

4 sticks of celery
½ cabbage
2 carrots

■ Wash all the vegetables. Cut them into juicer-sized pieces, juice, stir and drink immediately.
Rich in beta-carotene, calcium, magnesium, manganese, potassium, folic acid and vitamin C.
Traces of iron and zinc.

CELERY, WATERCRESS AND PEPPER

This pale green juice is pleasantly peppery – and another powerhouse of nutrients. It is deeply cleansing and an immune system booster said to be a protector against cancer, and is particularly beneficial for the skin. Said also to lower blood pressure, it improves circulation and alleviates migraine.

Small bunch of watercress
6 sticks of celery
1 yellow pepper

■ Wash all the vegetables. Cut them into juicer-sized pieces, juice, stir and drink immediately.
Rich in beta-carotene, folic acid, calcium, iron, magnesium, manganese, potassium, sodium and vitamins B, C and E.
Traces of B vitamins, copper and zinc.

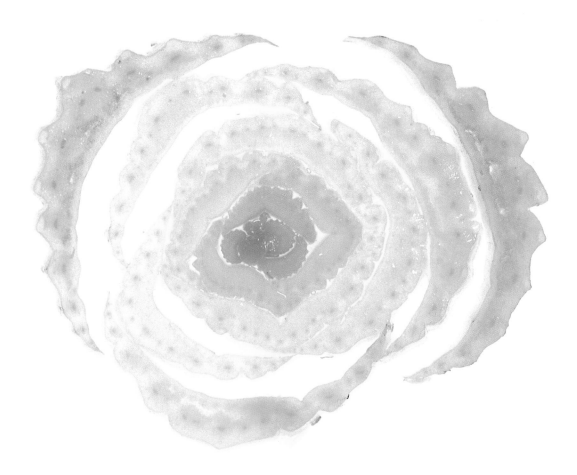

Lettuce

Lettuce is another strong green juice that needs to be diluted with other sweeter juices before it is drunk. It contains a lot of water and is highly diuretic, so useful for anyone with water retention. It also contains antioxidants and silicon, which protects the bones. Its calming properties make it beneficial as a late-night drink to aid peaceful sleep.

LETTUCE AND APPLE

This is a thin green juice that is energizing yet calming at the same time. It is deeply cleansing and the combination of parsley and apple sweeten one's

breath. However, it has a slightly bitter taste, so is best when made with a sweet apple. If, even then, it is still too bitter for you, use an extra apple.

1 small head of lettuce
1 apple
Large handful of parsley

■ Wash all the ingredients. Juice the parsley in batches between the apple and lettuce, as it is very fibrous and needs the other ingredients to help it through your juicer. Stir well and drink.
Rich in beta-carotene, folic acid, calcium, pectin, magnesium, potassium, phosphorus and vitamin C.

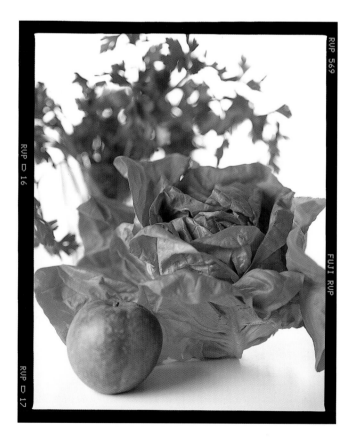

Traces of other B vitamins, copper and zinc.

LETTUCE AND TOMATO

All the nutrients of a salad in a drink! In spite of the murky green colour, this juice has a fresh, clean taste. Use a small lettuce or half an ordinary one.

1 small head of lettuce
(or ½ a normal lettuce)
2 tomatoes
2 handfuls of beansprouts

■ Wash all of the ingredients and cut into juicer-sized pieces. Stir well and drink the juice immediately.
Rich in beta-carotene, folic acid, vitamins C and E, calcium, magnesium, phosphorus, biotin, chlorine, potassium and sodium.
Traces of B vitamins, copper, zinc, iron and sulphur.

LETTUCE AND BEETROOT

A powerfully restorative juice, cleansing and strengthening for the whole system, it is particularly beneficial when drunk late at night. It promotes deep sleep and will aid the repair and renewal of cells during the night.

½ lettuce
2 beetroots

■ Wash the vegetables, then juice and drink immediately.
Rich in beta-carotene, folic acid, calcium, iron, sodium, potassium, phosphorus and vitamins B6 and C.
Traces of other B vitamins, copper and zinc.

Peppers

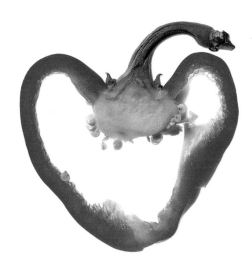

STRAIGHT PEPPER JUICE

Rather surprisingly, you can drink this juice neat, as it actually has a mild flavour. It is cleansing and energizing, stimulates the circulation and digestion, and normalizes blood pressure.

1 red pepper
1 yellow pepper

■ Wash, remove stalks and seeds, juice and drink.
Rich in beta-carotene, folic acid, calcium, magnesium, potassium and vitamin C.
Traces of B vitamins, vitamin E and iron.

PEPPER, SPINACH AND APPLE

A revitalizing juice with masses of antioxidants and health-protecting properties. The peppers and apples take away the bitterness of the spinach and watercress, and make this a pleasant juice to drink. This is said to be a cancer-fighting juice that normalizes blood pressure and reduces cholesterol.

2 sweet apples
1 red pepper
2 sticks of celery
1 large handful of spinach
1 large handful of watercress

■ Wash the ingredients and remove the stalk and seeds from the pepper. Juice each vegetable in rotation, stir and drink.
Rich in beta-carotene, folic acid, calcium, magnesium, iron, potassium, phosphorus, pectin and vitamins B3 and C.
Traces of other B vitamins, vitamin E, copper and zinc.

PEPPER AND GINGER

This is a deliciously spicy, peppery mix and a very startling yellow colour. An excellent detoxifier, it stimulates the digestion and the circulation, lowers blood pressure and guards against cancers and infections.

2 carrots
1 yellow pepper
1 thick slice of pineapple
½ inch ginger root

■ Remove the peel from the pineapple and ginger, and the yellow pepper's seeds. Wash the ginger, carrots and yellow pepper, then juice them. Stir the juice and drink it immediately.
Rich in beta-carotene, folic acid, calcium, magnesium, vitamin C, phosphorus and potassium.
Traces of B vitamins, vitamin E, zinc and iron.

PEPPERS AND ARTICHOKE

This recipe uses globe artichokes, which are renowned as diuretics and for their ability to cleanse the liver. This, along with the cleansing and toning effects of the parsley, makes this an effective juice for combating cellulite.

2 globe artichokes
2 red or yellow peppers
1 handful of parsley

■ Wash all the ingredients thoroughly and remove the stalks and seeds from the peppers. Juice the vegtables and herbs and drink immediately.
Rich in beta-carotene, folic acid, calcium, iron, magnesium, phosphorus, potassium, silica, sodium.
Traces of B vitamins, vitamin E and zinc.

PEPPERS AND CARROTS

This is a powerful antioxidant juice, and a superb detoxifier and energy booster. A mild diuretic and laxative, it is a good juice for a detoxification or juice fast (see page 100). It is also useful for fighting cystitis, PMS, headaches, migraines and promoting beautiful skin.

1 red or yellow pepper
6 lettuce leaves
1 large carrot

Rich in beta-carotene, folic acid, calcium, magnesium, phosphorus, potassium and vitamin C.
Traces of B vitamins, vitamin E, iron and zinc.

Spinach

Spinach is a perfect juice – immune system boosting, cancer-fighting and profoundly cleansing. Beneficial for a wide range of ailments, such as ulcers, anaemia, arthritis and fatigue, it has a strengthening effect upon the bones, teeth and gums. It also regulates the blood pressure and acts as a natural laxative. In spite of its powers, it must be used with caution; if used too frequently, it can have an over-intense cleansing effect. Because of its strong taste it should be mixed with something else.

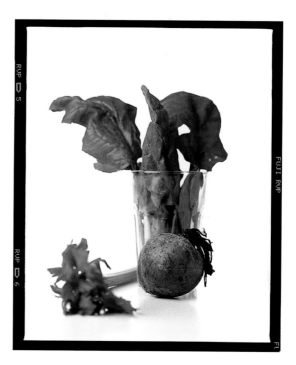

SPINACH, BEETROOT AND APPLE

This is a great booster for the immune system, and one of the best all-round cleansing and energizing health drinks. It also has a sensational taste – sweet because of the beetroot, but balanced by the spinach.

3 large handfuls of spinach
2 small beetroots
2 large apples

■ Wash all of the ingredients, being careful to leave any organic leaves on the beetroot for juicing. The spinach will be the toughest ingredient to juice, so put a little at a time into the juicer, followed by the beetroot or apple. Stir this very frothy juice and drink it immediately. If you wish, you can scoop off the top froth as it is not appealing to everyone!
Rich in beta-carotene, folic acid, calcium, iron, magnesium, phosphorus, potassium and vitamins B3, B6 and C.
Traces of copper and zinc.

SPINACH, CABBAGE AND ASPARAGUS

This protective, cleansing juice boosts the immune system. Asparagus is beneficial for the kidneys, and spinach cleanses the liver. It is mildly laxative and diuretic, and good for clearing the skin of spots.

½ cabbage
Large handful of spinach
6 sticks of asparagus

■ Wash and chop the vegetables to fit the juicer. Juice, stir and drink immediately.
Rich in beta-carotene, folic acid, calcium, iron, potassium and vitamins B3, B6, C and E.
Traces of zinc.

SPINACH, BEETROOT AND AVOCADO

This thin, purple and extremely powerful antioxidant, cleansing juice tastes predominantly of beetroot, meaning it is very sweet and takes the bite out of the spinach. Avocado doesn't really juice; it produces more of a pulp. However, it does add sweetness and a smooth texture to this juice and, nutritionally, protects the body against anaemia.

Large handful of spinach
Small handful of parsley
1 medium beetroot
1 stick of celery
1 avocado

■ Wash all the vegetables thoroughly under running water except the avocado, which should be peeled and then stoned. Leave all the leaves on the celery and beetroot, as these can be juiced, too. Alternate the vegetables which you put through the juicer, spacing the spinach and parsley, as their fibres can cause clogging. Stir and drink the juice immediately.
Rich in beta-carotene, folic acid, calcium, iron, manganese, potassium, sodium and vitamins B3, B6 and C.
Traces of zinc.

Turnip

Turnip produces a creamy, harmless-looking juice but, rather than being bland, it is actually deliciously peppery. It is best when combined with other sweeter vegetable juices, which takes away some of its bite. An excellent detoxification juice, it affects both the digestive system and the blood. Its high level of calcium is good for strengthening the bones and teeth, and its high potassium content makes its effect alkalizing, so that it reduces hyperacidity and generally cleanses the body.

■ TURNIP, CARROT AND DANDELION

Dandelions are one of the most useful weeds in the garden. The leaves are ideal for juicing and are packed with nutrients. Its French name of "pis-en-lit" provides a clue about its diuretic properties! This is a juice that builds up, cleanses and balances the body. If you find it too bitter, add extra carrots or a beetroot.

Handful of dandelion leaves
3 carrots
2 turnips

■ Scrub the turnips and carrots and leave on any top leaves, if organic. Wash the dandelion leaves and juice these first in batches, interspersed with other vegetables if they choke the juicer. Stir and drink the juice immediately.
Rich in beta-carotene, folic acid, vitamin C, calcium, magnesium, phosphorus and potassium.
Traces of B vitamins, iron and zinc.

■ TURNIP TONIC

This is a real super-juice if you are tired or under-the-weather. It is strengthening, an immune system booster, cleansing and an excellent all-round pick-me-up. Use it when you are under stress or are physically exhausted – or for jet lag. It has a deliciously peppery taste.

2 small turnips
2 beetroots
2 carrots
2 stalks of celery
Small bunch of watercress
1 apple

■ Wash and chop all of the ingredients, and juice in rotation. Stir and drink immediately.
Rich in beta-carotene, folic acid, iron, pectin, vitamin C, calcium, magnesium, phosphorus, potassium and manganese.
Traces of B vitamins, vitamin E, copper and zinc.

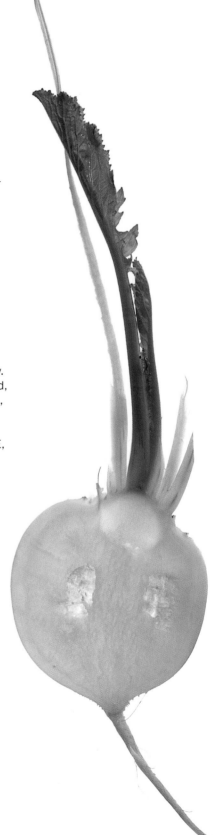

Cucumber

Cucumber is a great juicing vegetable because it produces so much liquid and its mild taste dilutes more bitter or peppery juices. It's a bit insipid on its own, but it has soothing qualities, particularly for the respiratory and digestive tracts, which makes it a very useful mixer with protective antioxidant juices. It is also cleansing, with both diuretic and laxative properties, and is beneficial for anyone suffering from kidney or bladder stones. Skin, nails and hair all also benefit.

CUCUMBER AND GINGER

This juice is both cleansing and stimulating. It is beneficial for menstrual pain and heavy periods, and particularly good for weak or brittle nails.

1 cucumber
½ inch ginger root

■ Wash, juice and drink immediately.
Rich in folic acid, vitamin C, calcium, beta-carotene, silica and potassium.
Traces of iron and zinc.

CUCUMBER, CARROT AND ROCKET

The strong, bitter flavour of rocket is sweetened by the carrots and cucumber. Rocket is a powerful antioxidant, but, if you can't find rocket, substitute watercress or spinach. This blend has a pleasant, mildly savoury taste. If you want a more peppery flavour (or more antioxidants), add more rocket. This mixture combats the build- up of uric acid, making it of benefit to anyone with rheumatism or kidney or bladder stones.

Large handful of rocket
2 medium carrots
½ cucumber

■ Wash the ingredients, leaving any organic leaves on the carrots. Juice and drink immediately.
Rich in beta-carotene, folic acid, vitamin C, calcium, magnesium, phosphorus, potassium, silica and sodium.
Traces of B vitamins, iron and zinc.

CUCUMBER, PARSLEY AND CARROT

This is both a health booster (because of the antioxidant effects of the parsley and carrots) and a diuretic (because of the parsley and the cucumber), all in one! Parsley juice is very strong, but its bitterness is alleviated by the carrots and cucumber.

4 large carrots
Large handful of parsley
½ cucumber

■ Wash all the ingredients thoroughly. Leave the cucumber and carrots unpeeled and the green tops on the carrots if organic. Cut them to fit the juicer. Put the parsley into the juicer first; if the herb is very fibrous, add it in batches, interspersing it with cucumber. Stir well and drink immediately.
Rich in beta-carotene, folic acid, vitamin C, calcium, magnesium, silica and potassium.
Traces of B vitamins, iron and zinc.

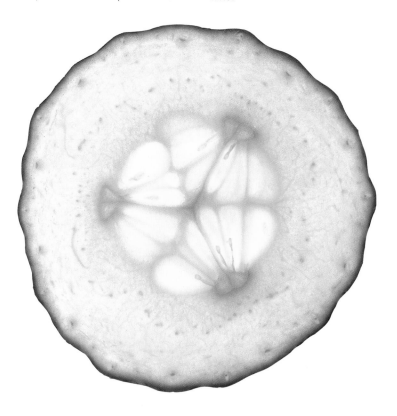

Chicory

Chicory juice is very bitter and so is only ever used as part of a mixture with other vegetables. It does, however, have highly beneficial immune system boosting properties, as it contains quantities of beta-carotene, as well as iron and potassium. There is also anecdotal evidence to suggest that it may promote good eyesight.

CHICORY, CARROT AND CELERY

This powerful, antioxidant juice is an excellent all-round health-protector. Chicory is particularly cleansing for the liver and the blood and, when combined with carrots' renowned reputation for improving night vision, is an aid to eyesight.

1 head of chicory
2 carrots
2 sticks of celery
Handful of parsley

■ Wash all of the ingredients, juicing them in rotation so that the parsley will go through the machine smoothly. Stir and drink the juice immediately.
Rich in beta-carotene, folic acid, calcium, iron, manganese, magnesium, potassium and vitamins B3 and C.
Traces of other B vitamins, iron and zinc.

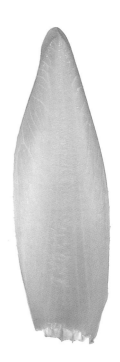

Celeriac

This is a delicious root vegetable. Its flavour is very nutty, rather than the celery-like taste that people often expect. It is high in antioxidants and a good diuretic and general cleanser. Of particular benefit to arthritis sufferers, it is also said to have a calming effect upon the nervous system.

CELERIAC AND WATERCRESS

The carrots and watercress add their own health-giving properties to this powerful antioxidant mix, making this a general health protector and detoxifier. It has a strong, peppery, slightly earthy taste, and the colour is decidedly murky – but it really is quite palatable. If you find it too strong, add extra carrots.

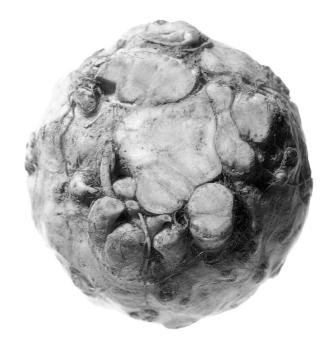

½ celeriac
Handful of watercress
2 carrots

■ Wash the ingredients, paying particular attention to the celeriac. Juice in rotation. Stir and drink the juice immediately.
Rich in beta-carotene, vitamin C, calcium, folic acid, magnesium, phosphorus and potassium.
Traces of B vitamins.

Onion

Unsurprisingly, onion juice has a strong flavour, so it is not something to drink by itself unless you want to bring tears to your eyes. It is, however, a wonderful immune system booster, and antibiotic. It is also a natural antiseptic and great detoxifier.

■ ONION, CELERIAC AND CUCUMBER

The celeriac's nutty flavour and the highly liquid cucumber dilute the onion's more overpowering effects. This juice is of particular benefit if you feel congested or you're trying to keep a cold at bay. If you want more sweetness, add another carrot.

½ celeriac
½ small onion
1 cucumber
2 carrots

■ Wash the celeriac, cucumber and carrots. Chop them into suitably-sized chunks to fit the juicer. Peel the onion. Juice each ingredient alternately – the celeriac will probably need to go through in small pieces, as it is so dense. Stir well and drink the juice immediately.
Rich in beta-carotene, folic acid, vitamin C, calcium, magnesium, phosphorus, chlorine, silica and potassium.
Traces of B vitamins, iron, copper and zinc.

■ ONION AND GRAPEFRUIT

It sounds like a curious mixture – and it does taste strange – but it works well for catarrh and hoarseness. It is also a powerful antioxidant.

2 large, sweet grapefruits
1 small onion

■ Peel the ingredients. Juice them and drink immediately.
Rich in beta-carotene, folic acid, vitamin C, calcium, magnesium, phosphorus, potassium and chlorine.
Traces of copper, iron, manganese, zinc and vitamins B and E.

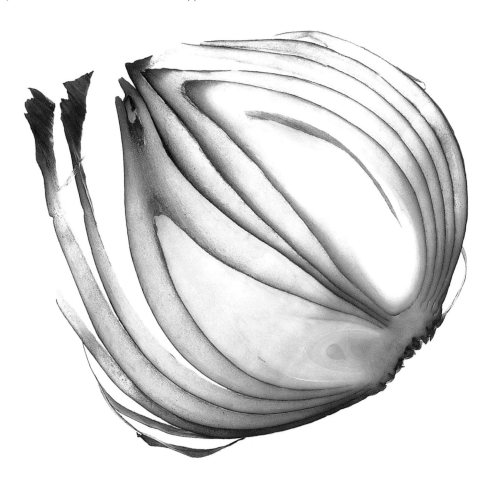

Fennel

Although too strong to drink alone, fennel has an unmistakable aniseed taste and is very good for pepping up other blander juices. It is used by naturopaths for nausea, menstrual and menopausal problems. Taken internally, it acts as a skin cleanser and so is excellent for spots and blemishes. It also strengthens the blood and is beneficial for weight loss.

FENNEL AND CUCUMBER

A light, refreshing juice that tastes like Pernod! If it's not sweet enough, add more carrot. This juice is ideal if you are

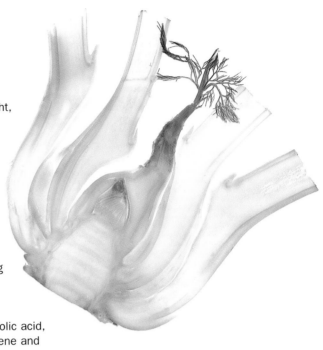

hoping to lose weight, and supports the immune system at the same time.

1 head of fennel
½ cucumber
2 carrots

■ Wash all the vegetables thoroughly under running water, then juice them. Stir and drink this immediately.
Rich in vitamin C, folic acid, calcium, beta-carotene and potassium.
Traces of B vitamins, iron and zinc.

Parsnip

Packed with B vitamins and vitamin E, the parsnip produces a very sweet juice. It strengthens nails, relieves bronchial problems, and is a good detoxifier, particularly for the kidneys, acting as a mild diuretic and laxative. Alone, it can be a bit too sweet, so it's best mixed with something spicy or peppery.

PARSNIP AND POTATO

By itself, the potato does not make a particularly appetizing juice, but it balances well with the sweetness of the parsnip and the peppery flavour of celery. A very useful source of vitamin C, especially in winter, the potato's antacid properties make it very soothing and cleansing for the digestive tract.

In fact, in naturopathic clinics, it is often used to treat ulcers. It is also a good beauty treatment for the skin.

2 potatoes
2 parsnips
3 sticks of celery

■ Wash all the vegetables and cut them into chunks to fit your juicer. Alternate root vegetables with the celery, as they are dense and quite hard to juice. If your juicer seems to be straining in the attempt, use smaller pieces. Juice, mix well and drink this immediately.
Rich in folic acid, calcium, magnesium, phosphorus, potassium, chlorine, manganese and vitamins B3, E and C.
Traces of other B vitamins, copper, iron and zinc.

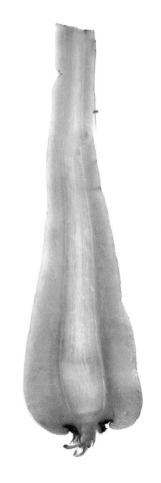

Garlic

This is not a juice to drink before you go to a party, or you may find that it's not only infections that give you a wide berth! However, the antibiotic, antibacterial, antiseptic and antiviral qualities of garlic make it a force to be reckoned with when it comes to health protection. It is said to protect against heart disease and cancer, and is second to none when it comes to fighting off a cold. You need only the tiniest amount for mixing with sweeter juices like carrot and beetroot.

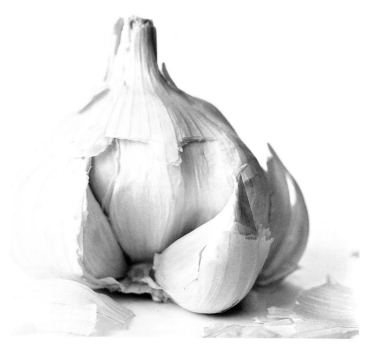

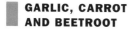 **GARLIC, CARROT AND BEETROOT**

This juice is the ultimate antioxidant cocktail and infection fighter. It is able to purify the blood, strengthen the heart and circulation, as well as lower cholesterol. If you drink it at the very first hint of a cold, you might be able to stop the cold straight away.

2 cloves of garlic
2 carrots
2 small beetroots
2 sticks of celery

■ Wash the vegetables and peel the garlic. Juice, and drink this immediately.
Rich in beta-carotene, folic acid, calcium, iron, magnesium, manganese, potassium and vitamins B6, C and E.
Traces of other B vitamins and zinc.

Sweet Potato

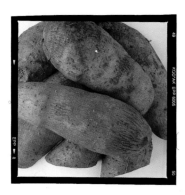

The juice of a sweet potato is not quite as horrible as that produced by the ordinary potato, but it is still better to drink it as part of a mix of other juices. Full of antioxidants and highly nutritious, it is very detoxifying (particularly for the digestive system) and stimulates circulation. It also is profoundly energizing and is said to be beneficial for ulcers and to guard against cancer.

■ **SWEET POTATO, LEEK AND CARROT**

This is a great antioxidant cocktail and so a good all-round health protector. Of particular benefit for relieving headaches, this juice is very cleansing and energizing.

1 large sweet potato
1 leek
2 carrots
2 sticks of celery

■ Wash all of the ingredients, juice them and drink this immediately.
Rich in beta-carotene, folic acid, calcium, magnesium, chlorine, phosphorus, potassium, sodium, and vitamins B3, C, E and K.
Traces of other B vitamins, sulphur, iron and zinc.

Radish

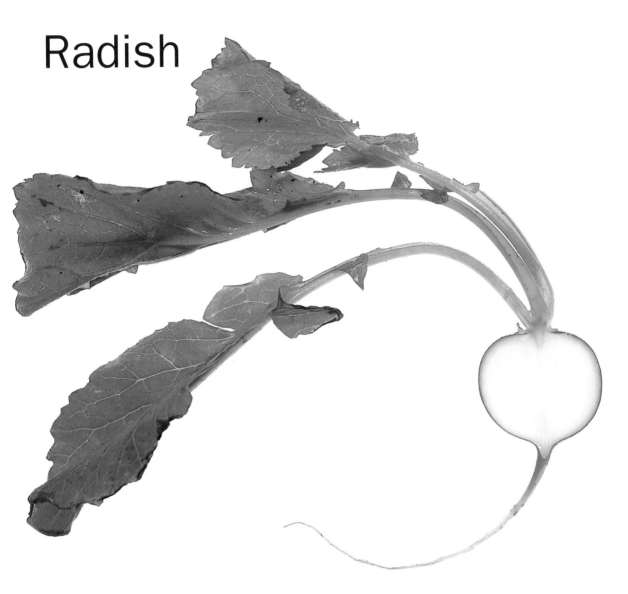

The radish produces a very strong peppery juice that is undrinkable unless diluted. It is deeply cleansing and a powerful antioxidant, therefore excellent as part of a detoxification plan. It particularly works on the respiratory system, clearing sinuses and fighting off infection, and stimulates the digestive system.

▍ RADISHES AND GREENS

This radish and cauliflower combination produces a fairly bitter, peppery taste which is sweetened by the addition of carrots and white cabbage. Don't use a green or red cabbage for this particular juice cocktail, or the taste will be far too strong. Cabbage is known to be good for clearing the skin of blemishes, while carrots are also known to improve skin conditions.

As well as being good for the skin, this highly protective juice is also good as an all-round immune system booster and is said to fight off infection very effectively.

6 radishes
½ small white cabbage
½ small cauliflower
2 carrots

■ Wash all of the vegetables thoroughly and juice them, alternating between each of the ingredients. Stir well and drink this juice immediately.
Rich in beta-carotene, folic acid, calcium, magnesium, potassium, iron and vitamins C, E and K.
Traces of B vitamins, sodium, sulphur and zinc.

PART 3

health

directory

Raw fruit and vegetable juices
provide a concentrated form of essential
vitamins and minerals, enzymes and sugars. Because
they are raw, they retain all the nutrients often destroyed by
cooking and, simply because they are juices, they are much easier to
take than if you were trying to consume the same amount of raw food.
Liquid literally slips into your system; it's a lot easier to drink a glass of

Juices
for ailments

carrot juice than to munch a pound of carrots! Juices are very nutritious and
wonderful cleansers of the body, but they can also be used for specific
therapeutic purposes and to help relieve unpleasant symptoms. Like
most natural remedies, they take time to work, but if you treat
juices the way people do vitamin pills – consuming
them every day – you should start to see
benefits within a few weeks.

Juices for
children

The fruit juices in this book are usually very appealing to children, since they are so sweet and delicious. In an age when most children are constantly targeted by advertisers to eat the least nutritious junk food, fresh juices are an easy way to ensure that they are taking in the vitamins and minerals they need to grow. Remember that most of the juices on the supermarket shelves have been there for some time, so even the "freshly squeezed" ones will have lost much of their nutritional value, while the other "juice drinks" will have had very little real juice to start with, as they are generally 90 per cent water, with sugar added to a little juice.

Most vegetable juices will not appeal to children, as their taste is too bitter and they are, in any case, too powerful for young bodies. Exceptions to this are the carrot and beetroot mixes, which are sweeter than most vegetable juices and can be given to children on an occasional basis.

As all too many parents know, it can be very difficult to persuade children to eat enough fruit and vegetables, and many children simply refuse to eat any at all. At this point, juices can become your salvation! Juices contain vital nutrients in a form that is usually extremely palatable to children.

Young children (under seven) should not have undiluted juice; add an equal amount of water to the juice. Give children aged seven to 14 half the amount of juice in the recipes, which are for adults. After the age of 14, children may drink the same amount, and strength, of juice as adults. Young children should have no more than one juice a day, but teenagers can have up to two glasses.

You can also add live natural yogurt or tofu to juices in order to turn them into smoothies (see page 41). This will also add protein to drinks. Simply juice as usual, then mix the juice with the yogurt or tofu in a blender or food processor.

Children tend to like the sweetest juices, of course. Particularly sweet ones are straight pear or apple juice, or those containing banana, mango or pawpaw, all of which provide extra energy for the body. Start your children on juices at an early age, and they will be healthier, less prone to infection, and have a good habit started for life.

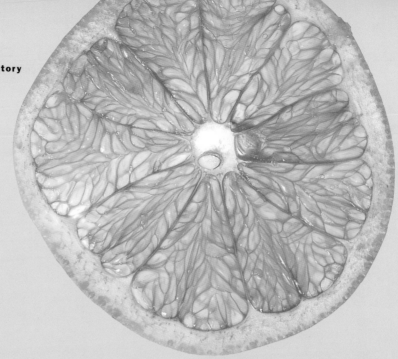

■ Acne

Blemishes are most commonly the result
of hormonal imbalance or a poor diet, or a
combination of the two. Acne is usually
associated with adolescence but blemishes
can occur at any time, and many women get
them just before menstruation whatever their
age. Cutting out junk foods and spices
and drinking plenty of water will help. To
counteract acne, take two to three glasses
a day of one of the following, varying the
juices regularly:

Berries and cherries (page 65)
Broccoli and beetroot (page 68)
Carrot and apple (page 66)
Orange and grapefruit (page 58)
Spinach, carrot and asparagus (page 74)

■ Anaemia

Iron deficiency anaemia frequently occurs
among women who suffer from heavy periods
or do not have enough iron (and possibly folic
acid) in their diets. It will help to include more
red meat and liver in the diet and one to two
of the following juices every day. Vary the
juices regularly:

Apricot and kiwi (page 50)
Blackberry and watermelon (page 47)

Broccoli and beetroot (page 68)
Grapes and plums (page 53)
Spinach, beetroot and avocado (page 74)

■ Anti-ageing

Vitamins A (beta-carotene in fruit and
vegetables), C and E, together with the
minerals zinc and selenium, are prime
antioxidants. Once taken into the body, they
act as soldiers against free radicals, which
are electrochemically unbalanced molecules
generated within our bodies by such things as
pollution, cigarettes, pesticides, drugs,
overeating, stress and certain foods.

These free radical molecules are
responsible on a cellular level for many of the
degenerative diseases associated with
ageing. They react with other, healthy
molecules, making them unstable too, thus
starting a chain reaction of cellular
destruction. This can lead to serious
degenerative conditions such as cancer and
heart disease, but also to other signs of
premature ageing, such as wrinkes and the
loss of muscle strength. Most of the recipes
in this book contain antioxidants which fight
against this process. Drinking as many
different juices as possible will give you the
best protection. Drink at least one a day, but
preferably two or three, of the following:

Berries and cherries (page 65)
Carrot and apple (page 66)
Herby carrot (page 66)
Orange and grapefruit (page 58)
Pawpaw and ginger (page 51)

■ Arthritis and rheumatism

Rheumatism is the lay term for pain and stiffness in the muscles and joints, while arthritis refers to pain and swelling in the joints. Osteoarthritis, a degenerative disease of the joints, wears away the protective cartilage of the fingers, knees, hips and spine. Severe pain and swelling may occur, which can lead to immobility.

Certain juices have anti-inflammatory effects, and these can therefore help to reduce swelling and the consequent pain and immobility. These include artichoke, carrot, celery and beetroot juice. Pineapple juice may also be helpful. Drink one glass of the following twice a day, and remember to vary the juices:

Beetroot and cucumber (page 67)
Celeriac and watercress (page 77)
Cherry and nectarine (page 53)
Cucumber, carrot and rocket (page 76)
Spinach, beetroot and apple (page 74)

■ Asthma

Asthma may be caused by allergic reactions, airborne pollutants, anxiety and cold air; there are different triggers for different people. Often, relaxation and breathing techniques can be beneficial, and various juices, like those below, can help to soothe the asthmatic cough.

Banana and cranberry (page 61)
Berries and cherries (page 65)
Broccoli and beetroot (page 68)
Lettuce and tomato (page 72)

■ Bad breath

Bad breath is usually a symptom of another underlying problem, such as poor digestion or constipation, although it can also be caused by tooth decay or gum disease. If it is the latter, it is obviously vital to consult a dentist. If the former, drink one of the following each morning and night, varying the juices:

Cabbage, quince and carrot (page 69)
Herby carrot (page 66)
Lettuce and apple (page 72)

■ Cancer protection

Different types of cancer can be triggered in different people by different causes. However,

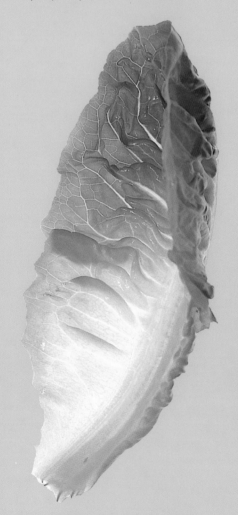

there are some safeguards that everyone should adopt – not smoking, using sun protection and eating a healthy diet. It is in the last category that juices can help, as they provide such a powerhouse of antioxidants (see *Anti-ageing* on page 86). Drink one to three glasses a day of the following juices, changing them often:

All-currant cocktail (page 49)
Broccoli and beetroot (page 68)
Cabbage and celery (page 69)
Pawpaw, pineapple and mango (page 51)

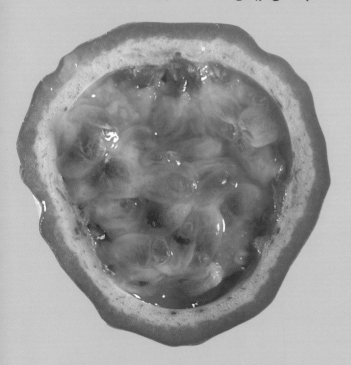

Pepper, spinach and apple (page 73)
Strawberry and redcurrant (page 65)
Sweet potato, leek and carrot (page 80)

■ Cellulite

Although still dismissed as an invention of the beauty trade, most women agree that there is a difference between cellulite and fat. Cellulite is dimpled fat that tends to appear on certain areas of women's bodies, notably the thighs, buttocks, upper arms and abdomen. It is usually a sign that the lymphatic system is not carrying toxins out of the body efficiently; both skin brushing and regular exercise will help the condition. Also, the following juices will be beneficial, if drunk on a daily basis and varied frequently:

Cucumber, parsley and carrot (page 76)
Peppers and artichoke (page 73)
Spinach, carrot and asparagus (page 74)
Turnip, carrot and dandelion (page 75)

■ Cholesterol

A diet containing too much saturated fat will produce an excess of cholesterol in the body. This can build up along the walls of the arteries and result in atherosclerosis. Cholesterol is linked with heart disease and also with gallstones and cellulite. Saturated fats are found in red meat, dairy products and fried food, and are best avoided. The following juices promote the health of the arteries. Drink one a day, varying them frequently.

Garlic, carrot and beetroot (page 80)
Orange and grapefruit (page 58)
Pineapple, banana and apple (page 62)
Tomato and celery (page 70)

■ Circulation

One of the most obvious signs of poor circulation is having cold hands and feet. The most valuable thing you can do to remedy this is to exercise regularly, even if it is just walking several times a day. Stopping smoking and lowering your salt intake will also help. Strong foods spiced with things like garlic and ginger revive sluggish circulation. These can be incorporated into your normal diet and also in juices. Drink one or two of these every day, alternating often:

Apple, pineapple and ginger (page 46)
Garlic, carrot and beetroot (page 80)

Straight mandarin juice (page 59)
Pepper and ginger (page 73)

■ Constipation

Regular daily juicing should eradicate
constipation as a matter of course. However,
regular exercise, a sensible diet and, above
all, plenty of water, will be beneficial, too.
Apple is very effective for any digestive
problem, and most dark-green vegetables
stimulate the bowel. However, many juices
act as intestinal brooms. Drink two to three
a day of the following, varying the juices for
the best effect:

Apple, orange and pineapple (page 46)
Carrot and apple (page 66)
Pear and pineapple (page 48)
Straight pepper juice (page 73)
Plum, apple and fig (page 63)
Spinach, carrot and asparagus (page 74)

■ Cooling

When the body gets overheated (from very hot
weather or overexertion), one of the best
ways to cool it down is with celery juice. This
has the effect of not only normalizing the
body's temperature, but also replenishing
sodium, which is very useful if you have been
perspiring. Drink one of the following every
two or three hours:

Celery, cabbage and carrot (page 71)
Celery, watercress and pepper (page 71)
Tomato and celery (page 70)

■ Coughs and colds

You can help to ward off cold infections by a
daily glass or two of immune system boosting
juices. At the sign of the first symptom, drink
up to four glasses a day of the following
juices; those with onion or garlic are
particularly useful at this point, and can even

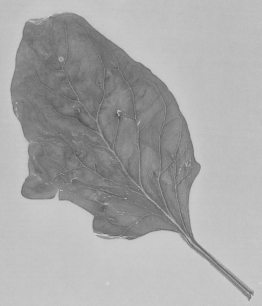

stop the infection in its tracks. (See also
Sore Throats on page 96.)

Carrot and apple (page 66)
Beetroot and carrot (page 67)
Garlic, carrot and beetroot (page 80)
Onion, celeriac and cucumber (page 78)
Orange and grapefruit (page 58)
Spinach, cabbage and asparagus (page 74)
Watercress and carrot (page 70)

■ Cramp

Cramp may be caused by a lack of certain
minerals such as potassium and magnesium.
Blackcurrant, passion fruit and melon are all
high in these two vital minerals. Banana is
another well-known cramp cure. To alleviate
this condition, drink one or two glasses a day
of one of the following:

Banana and melon (page 61)
Blackberry and watermelon (page 47)
Melon and grape (page 56)

■ Cystitis

Cystitis can be a painful and distressing
problem. Not only does it make you want to

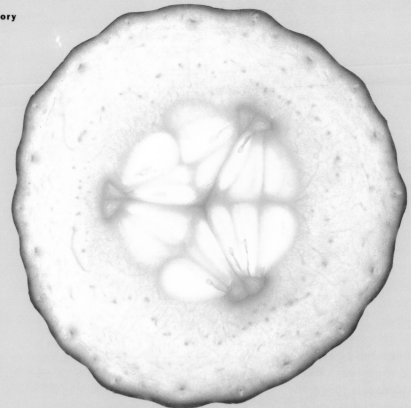

rush to the bathroom every few minutes, there is an excruciating burning when you get there. It is caused by an inflammation of the lining of the bladder, and this should be flushed out with as much water as possible, plus one or two of the following juices daily, in rotation:

Banana and cranberry (page 61)
Peppers and carrots (page 73)
Turnip, carrot and dandelion (page 75)

■ Detoxification

Many of the juices in this book are deeply cleansing and, whether taken on a regular basis or as part of a juice fast (see pages 100–123), will help to rid the body of toxins so that it can repair and rejuvenate. Some of the best are:

Cabbage and sweet potato (page 69)
Carrot and apple (page 66)
Celeriac and watercress (page 77)
Kiwi cocktail (page 54)

Orange and banana (page 58)
Spinach, beetroot and avocado (page 74)

■ Diarrhoea

Diarrhoea can result from a variety of causes from parasites, food poisoning and stress to jet lag. If it continues, always consult your doctor. In the meantime, abstain from food, drink as much water as you can, and one or two of the following juices:

Apple juice, diluted half and half with still filtered water (page 46)
Carrot juice, diluted half and half with still filtered water (page 66)
After symptoms start to diminish: Plum and pineapple (page 63)

■ Eczema and psoriasis

These skin ailments are widespread and can have a variety of causes, including stress, allergic reaction, heredity and fatigue. A warm bath with a soothing oil such as camomile, lavender or geranium is very beneficial. If the problem is triggered by stress or fatigue, plenty of rest and relaxation exercises are also recommended. Drink one or two of the following pure, cleansing juices daily:

Straight apple juice (page 46)
Apricot and kiwi (page 50)
Mango cocktail (page 55)
Straight pear juice (page 48)

■ Energy boosters

These juices work whether you are suffering from a feeling of constant weariness or simply want to raise your general energy levels. Bear in mind that you need rest as well if you are to maintain high energy levels, and a poor diet with lots of junk food, fat, sugar and salt will deplete your stores of energy. Drink two to three of the following juices daily, varying them frequently:

Straight apple juice (page 46)
Blackberry and watermelon (page 47)
Carrot and kiwi (page 66)
Grape, pineapple and apricot (page 53)
Lettuce and apple (page 72)
Orange and carrot (page 58)

■ Eyes

The old wives' tale about carrots helping you to see in the dark is based on fact, after all! Carrots contain carotenoids that protect the eyes, as do several other fruits and vegetables. For general eye health (especially if you spend your life staring at a computer) try one of these daily, alternating the juices often for the best effects.

Broccoli and beetroot (page 68)
Chicory, carrot and celery (page 77)
Herby carrot (page 66)
Mango cocktail (page 55)

■ Fever

Naturopaths regard fever as a good sign; the body is raising its temperature to kill off invading bacteria that can't stand the heat. While fever can be dangerous if prolonged, lowering the temperature before it has finished its job also means that the infection is all too likely to recur. You should always consult a doctor in cases of serious fever, especially in children. However, if it is a relatively mild accompaniment to flu, the best remedy is to retire to bed, drink as much

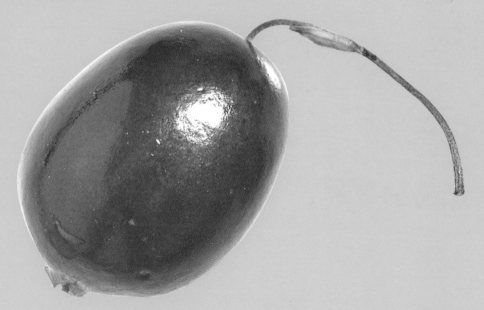

water as you can and up to three of the following juices daily, rotating them often:

Straight pear juice (page 48)
Straight pineapple juice (page 62)
Strawberry and redcurrant (page 65)

■ Flatulence

Flatulence is a sign that the digestive system is functioning poorly. Herbal teas like peppermint, fennel and ginger are often soothing. It also may help to avoid mixing starch and protein at the same meal. The following juices are all soothing and restorative to the digestive tract. Drink one or two a day, often varying the kind you have.

Cabbage, quince and carrot (page 69)
Cucumber and ginger (page 76)
Fennel and cucumber (page 79)
Pawpaw and ginger (page 51)

■ Gallstones

Gallstones are gravel-like deposits in the gall bladder – usually caused by a diet that is too high in fat. There may be no symptoms for a

long time, or only mild ones, such as indigestion or feeling bloated, which are triggered by a very fatty meal. The obvious advice is to cut out fat as much as possible. The following juices, taken once a day, will also help:

Straight beetroot juice (page 67)
Pawpaw and ginger (page 51)
Radishes and greens (page 81)

■ Hair

The hair on your head is actually dead matter, but the root is alive. The following juices supply the vitamins and minerals necessary for healthy hair. Drink one a day, varying daily.

Berries and cherries (page 65)
Cabbage and sweet potato (page 69)
Mango cocktail (page 55)

■ Headache and migraine

Headaches are a result of various factors, including stress, poor diet or digestive

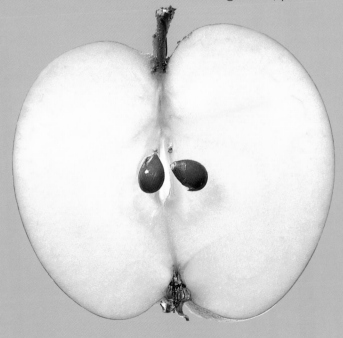

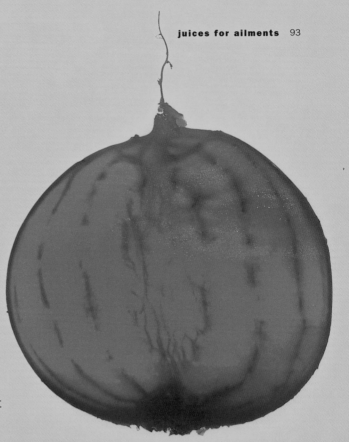

functioning, hormonal imbalance, allergies or tiredness. If you suffer from recurrent headaches, it is advisable to consult your doctor. Massaging the temples with lavender oil can ease a mild headache. Try the following juices, drinking up to three of them a day to combat headaches, alternating them frequently:

Cherry and nectarine (page 53)
Peppers and carrots (page 73)
Sweet potato, leek and carrot (page 80)

■ High blood pressure

Stress, smoking and high consumption of alcohol, salt and fat all contribute to high blood pressure, as do drinking coffee and tea. If you suffer from high blood pressure, it is advisable to change your diet in order to avoid these culprits as much as possible, and to also take measures to overcome stress, such as learning to meditate and using relaxation techniques. One of the following cleansing and soothing juices daily may also be beneficial:

Beetroot and cucumber (page 67)
Garlic, carrot and beetroot (page 80)
Tomato and celery (page 70)

■ Immune system boosters

Your resistance to infection and disease is increased by boosting your supply of antioxidants (see *Anti-ageing* on page 86). Most of the juices in this book are full of antioxidants, and drinking two or three of them on a regular daily basis is a good way of safeguarding your health. Some of the best are:

Beetroot and carrot (page 67)
Cabbage and sweet potato (page 69)
Carrot and apple (page 66)

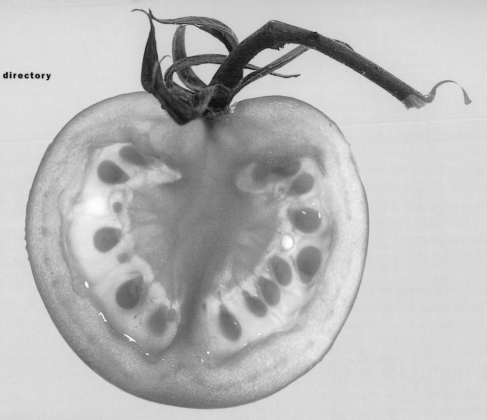

Onion, celeriac and cucumber (page 78)
Radishes and greens (page 81)
Straight tomato juice (page 70)
Turnip tonic (page 75)
Watercress and carrot (page 70)

■ Indigestion

Juices work particularly well on digestive problems of all kinds. Apple is very effective, especially when combined with thick, sweet, soothing juices such as mango, pawpaw, peach and pineapple. Drink up to three of the following juices every day:

Straight apple juice (page 46)
Parsnip and potato (page 79)
Pawpaw, pineapple and mango (page 51)
Raspberry and quince (page 64)

■ Insomnia

If your insomnia is caused by stress, try to take up some form of relaxation technique or meditation. It often helps to have a warm bath with lavender oil added before bedtime. Try to have a quiet time before you go to bed in order to allow yourself to wind down. The following juices are all naturally relaxing and

sleep-inducing. Drink one half an hour before going to bed.

Banana and cranberry (page 61)
Lettuce-based juices (page 72)
Raspberry and apple (page 64)

■ Kidney stones

If you have kidney stones, try to drink as much still, filtered water as you can in order to flush out the kidneys. The following juices help to cleanse the kidneys and dissolve stones in them. Drink two to three daily, alternating them.

Banana and cranberry (page 61)
Beetroot and spinach (see page 67)
Cucumber, carrot and rocket (page 76)
Peach and persimmon (page 57)

■ Nails

Many people suffer from brittle nails that break or tear easily, or grow with ridges and marks. The vitamins and minerals in most juices will help to alleviate these problems if they are drunk on a daily basis. However, these two juices will particularly help:

Cucumber and ginger (page 76)
Straight pawpaw juice (page 51)

■ Nausea

Nausea may be caused by a reaction to
something in your diet, for example fatty
foods, alcohol, morning sickness during
pregnancy or travel sickness. Ginger is
extremely calming as a tea or when mixed in
juices. Try:

Apple, pineapple and ginger (page 46)
Cucumber and ginger (page 76)

■ Periods

These juices are soothing for cramps and
also help to replace the iron lost if you have
heavy periods and lose a lot of blood. An
aromatherapy oil which I have found to be
very soothing for cramps is five drops each of
camomile and geranium oil mixed with 15
drops of clary sage oil into 2oz of carrier oil
(such as almond or grapeseed). Very gently,
massage this with the flat of your hand into
the abdomen, using a circular clockwise
motion. Also, drink two or three per day of the
following juices while symptoms persist:

Cucumber and ginger (page 76)
Apple, pineapple and ginger (page 46)
Apricot and pineapple (page 50)
Raspberry and quince (page 64)
Melon and plum (page 56)

■ PMS

The symptoms that women suffer from
vary greatly and include bloating, weight gain,
mood swings and cramps. The following juices
should help with water retention and cramps,
and have a general calming effect, too.
Drink two to three of the juices overleaf a
day, varying them regularly while symptoms
of PMS continue:

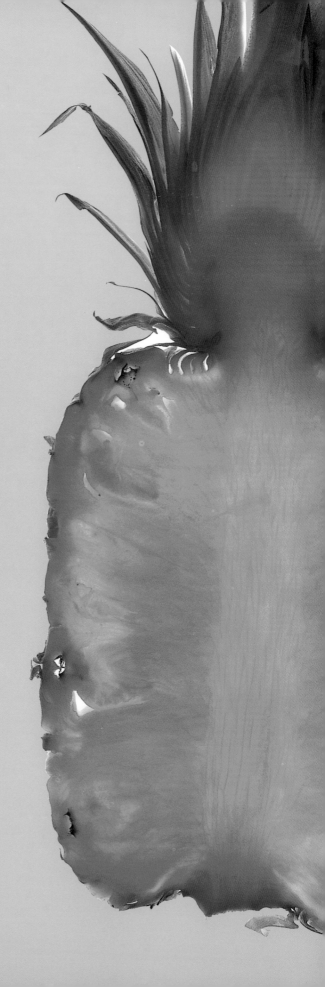

Apple, pineapple and ginger (page 46)
Peppers and carrots (page 73)
Sweet potato, leek and carrot (page 80)

■ Skin

Regularly drinking cleansing, antioxidant juices will benefit your appearance just as much as your internal health. The results show in your skin very quickly, particularly if you start off with a juice fast – when fine lines and blemishes seem to disappear and your skin takes on a healthy bloom. Drink one to three of the following juices every day, rotating them frequently:

Cabbage and sweet potato (page 69)
Straight cherry juice (page 53)
Mango cocktail (page 55)
Parsnip and potato (page 79)
Peppers and carrots (page 73)

■ Sore throat

Sore throats will often occur as one of the symptoms of a cold or respiratory infection. Try to rest quietly and drink one to three a day of the following juices, varying them often:

Celery, cabbage and carrot (page 71)
Onion and grapefruit (page 78)
Watercress and carrot (page 70)

■ Stress

Stress seems to be an unavoidable part of contemporary living, but over prolonged periods of time it undermines our general health to a marked degree. If you feel very stressed, try to do some form of relaxation or meditation, and make sure that you get enough rest. The following juices are calming and also help to restore the nutrients lost when we are under too much stress. Drink

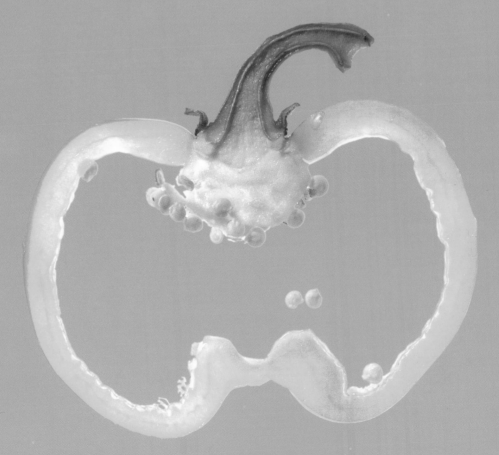

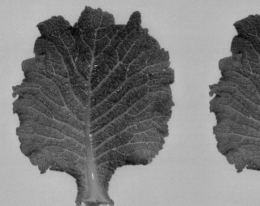
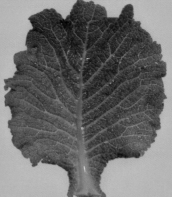
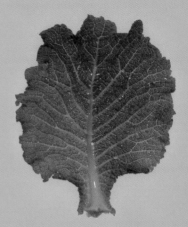

one to three of these a day, changing them as suggested before:

Celeriac and watercress (page 77)
Pear and banana (page 48)
Turnip tonic (page 75)
Watermelon and blackberries (page 60)

■ Ulcers

Ulcers are often a result of stress, and if this is your underlying problem, try to deal with it as above, as well as using the juices below. Potato, sweet potato and banana all help to soothe stomach ulcers. Drink one or two glasses of these juices every day, varying them as much as you can:

Parsnip and potato (page 79)
Pear and banana (page 48)
Sweet potato, leek and carrot (page 80)

■ Water retention

Water, or fluid, retention is an on-going problem for some people, but for most women, it occurs just before or during menstruation. Drinking plenty of water and avoiding tea and coffee help, as do gentle rhythmic exercises. There are plenty of diuretic juices you can drink also. One to three of the following should be drunk daily, frequently alternating the kind taken:

Apricot and kiwi (page 50)
Carrot and kiwi (page 66)
Cucumber, parsley and carrot (page 76)
Herby carrot (page 66)
Melon and grape (page 56)
Raspberry and melon (page 64)
Turnip, carrot and dandelion (page 75)
Watermelon and blackberries (page 60)

■ Weight loss

If you are overweight, the best way to lose weight is with a sensible, healthy, controlled diet. Crash diets don't work in the long-term, as you will pile the lost pounds back on as soon as you stop dieting. It is much better to lose weight gradually. A one or three-day juice fast is a great way to start, as you will not only lose some of your unwanted weight, but you will look and feel better, too, which is a great incentive to keep going. Drinking one to three juices a day is of great benefit, as it will give you a good nutritional basis for your diet, and the juices themselves are quite filling – a much better way to snack than a bar of chocolate! Any cleansing juices will work well for this purpose, but remember that you should vary them constantly in order to obtain the best supply of nutrients. Three good ones are:

Broccoli and beetroot (page 68)
Fennel and cucumber (page 79)
Straight pear juice (page 48)

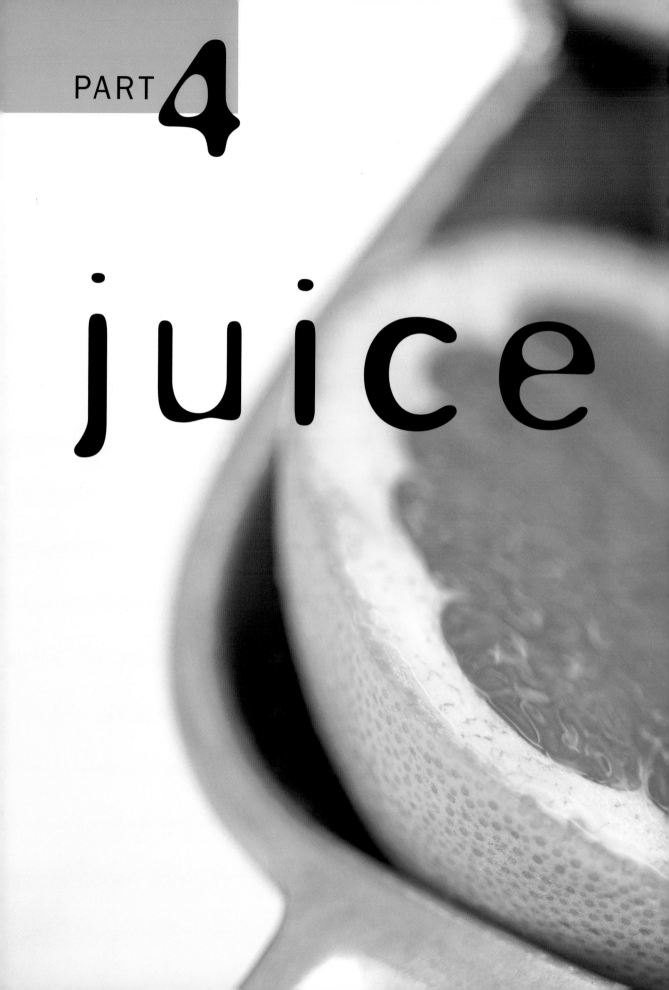

juice

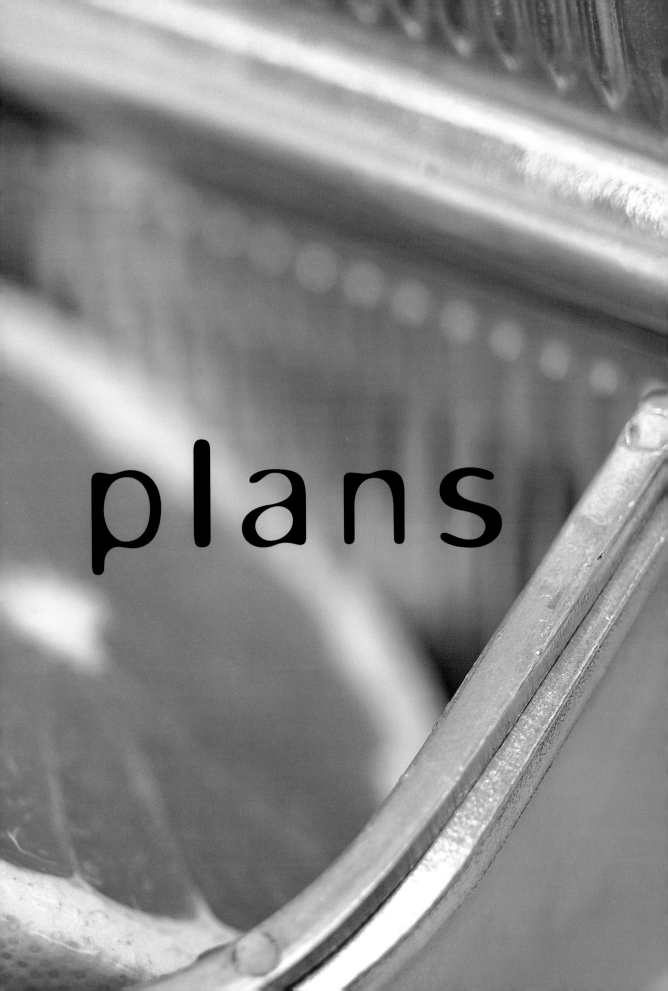
plans

Fasting is the oldest form of healing known to man, and is based on the simple premise that it gives the body time to heal itself during a period of abstinence from food. Perhaps the idea originated when early people watched how animals abstained from food when they were ill, and returned to it when they felt better.

Juice

Maybe, at a time when life was lived closer to nature, we instinctively fasted. Hippocrates and Plato recommended fasting, and most of the world's great religions advocate a period for it every year. In more recent times, juice fasts have been the basis of health cures in Europe, particularly since the nineteenth century. Some Germans, for instance, swear by the Rohsafte-Kur (the raw juice cure), claiming it is an effective way of detoxifying and restoring health to the body after excessive self-indulgence, periods of stress and fatigue, or illness. While such cures go on for a sustained period at a health clinic, even one day of juice fasting can have a remarkable effect, especially if you do it regularly. Juice fasting is one of the most cleansing and rejuvenating treatments you can have. During a fast, the body expels long-standing toxins. Its own

fasting

regulating mechanisms call upon the tissues in reverse order of their importance in the body, so that dead and diseased tissues and nutritional stores (or fat) are eliminated first. The body's in-built sense of priorities protects the major organs, accelerating its healing and cleansing processes and speeding up the proliferation of new, healthy cells. You can expect visible results, including improved skin tone, with fine lines disappearing and a bloom coming into the skin, silky soft hair and bright, clear eyes.

The one-day plan is an ideal way to dip your toe into the sea of juice fasting. You will no doubt already have been drinking juices regularly before you try this, but you may still feel a little nervous about the idea. However, virtually everyone feels better after a day of juice fasting, and the only people who should not try it are the frail or elderly, children, pregnant women, or people with eating disorders. Just about everybody else will benefit without adverse consequences. After all, many of the diseases of the modern world are caused by eating too much of the wrong foods,

The one-day plan

while fasting has repeatedly shown to lead to a longer and healthier life in animals. Still, it is not advisable to launch straight into a juice fast from your normal diet. You will need at least one day of preparation. Breaking the fast is equally important (see page 120); it is imperative not to rush back to old bad habits as soon as you have finished! The best time to fast is when you can focus on what you are doing, so a quiet weekend at home is ideal. Buy everything you need for juicing the day before you start. Fasting is a time for relaxing, not running around a supermarket.

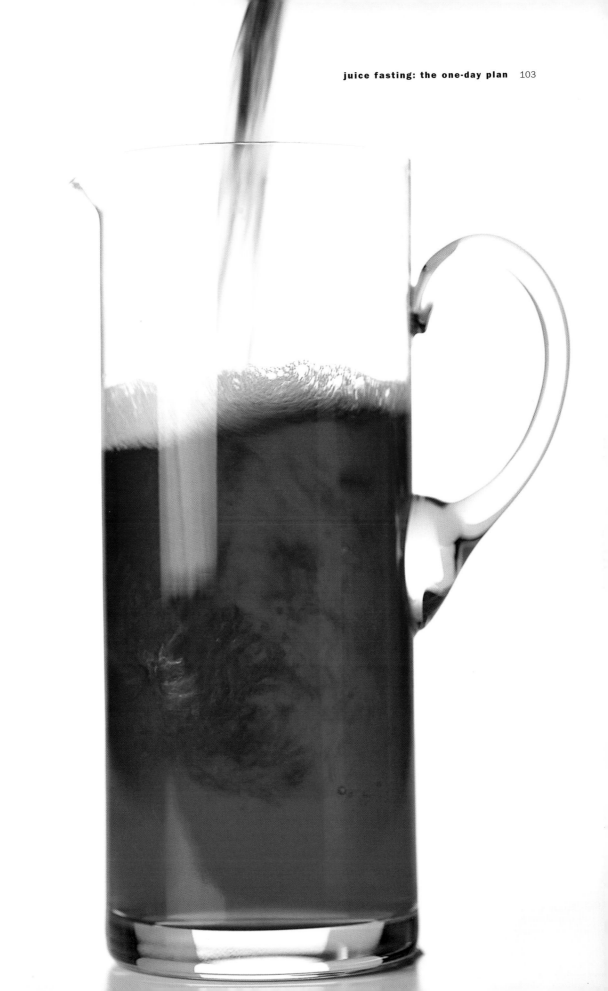

Preparation **day**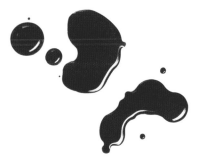

Before you start the juice fast itself, you need one or two days of dietary preparation. These are not difficult to arrange, even if you are not at home; you can easily replace a lunchtime sandwich with a salad. If you are away from your juicer most of the day, then adjust the times for your juices slightly so that you have one just before you leave the house, and one upon your return.

The purpose of this day or days is to prepare your body for the juice fast, and start the process of cleansing. You will need to increase your water intake dramatically. You should drink at least three pints of water (and preferably four) on top of any juices. Your diet for the preparation day or days should be high in raw fruit and vegetables, and a possible menu could look like this:

	Menu
Breakfast	■ When you first wake up, drink a cup of hot water to flush out the kidneys. Half an hour later, have breakfast. Choose from natural (live, preferably organic) yogurt (sweetened with a teaspoon of honey if you wish), with pumpkin, sesame and sunflower seeds, or a slice of wholemeal toast spread with honey. Have a piece of fruit and a cup of herbal tea (see page 105).
Mid-morning	■ A large glass of carrot and apple juice.
Lunch	■ This is your main meal. Make a salad (it can be as big as you like) from any of the following: beetroot, carrots, celery, chicory, cucumber, lettuce, peppers, radishes, spinach, spring onions, watercress and any other salad leaves. Dress with olive oil and lemon juice, with some black pepper and/or herbs. Serve with two pieces of wholemeal bread.
Mid-afternoon	■ Carrot and apple juice.
Supper	■ This works along the same principles as lunch, but this time it's as much fruit as you like. Eat fruits individually or make a big fruit salad and use apple juice to sweeten it. You can have yogurt with it, if you wish, or sweeten it further with honey.

If you feel hungry, eat fruit or vegetables as a snack, or make an extra juice (juice is surprisingly filling). Remember to drink your water quota (hot or cold), but, if you choose the latter, drink still rather than carbonated water.

DEEP CLEANSING

It is also a good idea to try out some other detoxifying treatments on these preparation days. Saunas and steam baths are particularly good, as they are highly detoxifying, but not really suitable for the fast day itself, as you may find yourself feeling a little dizzy or light-headed while fasting, and heat can exacerbate this. Ideally, you would spend the evening before you fast exercising, swimming and having some heat treatments, if you have a health club where you can do this. If you are feeling very tired or stressed, though, the best treatment is simply to rest.

HERBAL TEAS

Green and herbal teas contain no black tea, and, therefore, no caffeine or tannin to interfere with the cleansing process. They are very simple to make and a very good way to boost your liquid intake if you become bored with drinking plain water all of the time. You can choose from the array of herbal tea bags available in health food stores and supermarkets, or make your own by steeping a handful of herbs in boiling water for five minutes. Here are a few of my favourites:

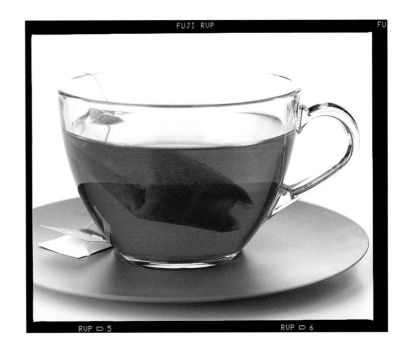

Camomile	■ Very soothing, particularly to the nervous and digestive systems, and also on an emotional level; it eases anxiety, headaches, insomnia, cystitis and water retention. Add honey if the taste is too bland for you.
Ginger	■ General stimulant excellent for respiratory (colds, coughs, flu, sore throats) and most digestive problems, poor circulation, fever and flatulence.
Peppermint	■ General pick-me-up and very good for soothing the digestion, relieving headaches and clearing mucus problems.

The one-day
juice fast

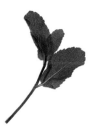

This is a day when you will be focusing on yourself only. You will probably find that what you want most is to be quiet and undisturbed, so, don't make any social plans and just take things as they come.

People have different reactions to juice fasting. You may feel great all day or experience one of the side effects that can occur, particularly if you have a big toxic build-up in your system or are very tired and under stress before you begin. If you do have any undesirable side effects, see the advice on side effects in the Three-Day Plan (page 113). The main thing you must do is take the day as it comes and do whatever you feel. Let your body call the shots today.

While the detoxification process is under way, you may feel tired. This may happen simply because you've slowed down for the day. If you do feel tired, just enjoy relaxing. But remember, this is not the time to take to your bed for the day, as some gentle exercise will be beneficial to this process of deep internal cleansing. As a guide, a fasting day should be planned like this; however, don't worry if you sleep late and it starts a little later. Fasting is also a time for relaxation. Above all else it should be a day you enjoy.

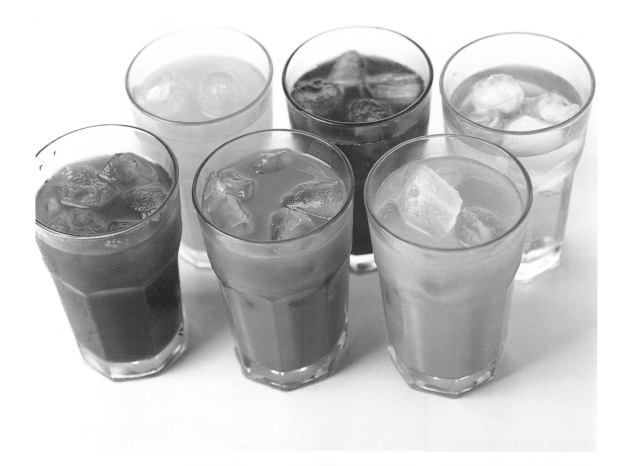

Time	Menu
8am	■ When you first wake up, drink a cup of hot water to flush out the kidneys (this and all drinks should be around 250ml [half a pint]). Half an hour later, have your first juice of the day. Carrot and apple is a good one, as it is so cleansing. Alternatively, choose a citrus fruit to wake you up.
8.30am	■ Before your shower, try dry skin brushing. This stimulates the circulation and the lymphatic system, and this, in turn, promotes the clearing of toxins (see page 108).
9.30am	■ Have a large glass of water or herbal tea.
10am	■ This is a good time to exercise, although not too vigorously. Yoga or walking is ideal, particularly if you are walking in a pleasant environment. This will also help to prevent a headache, which is a potential side effect on a juice fast.
11.30am	■ Have a large glass of water or herbal tea.
12.30pm	■ The second juice of the day and, as a replacement for lunch, this should be a substantial vegetable one, with beetroot, pepper, spinach or turnip in it.
1pm	■ Have another large glass of water or herbal tea. You may experience an energy dip now. If so, you can give in to it gracefully and have a nap or, if you prefer, go for a walk or do some simple stretching or yoga exercises. Relax afterwards for at least half an hour.
2.30pm	■ Have another large glass of water or herbal tea.
4pm	■ The third juice of the day. Boost blood sugar levels with apricot, pineapple, pawpaw, mango, cherry and nectarine juices.
5pm	■ Another large glass of water or herbal tea.
7.30pm	■ The fourth and last juice of the day — this one should be calming. Choose from banana, cranberry, watermelon, lettuce and apple juices.
9.30pm	■ Time for the last glass of water or herbal tea of the day. However, if you think this will wake you up in the night to go to the lavatory have it earlier, or skip it altogether. A good night's sleep is more important.
10pm	■ Have a relaxing bath with some aromatherapy oils (see page 108) and an early night.

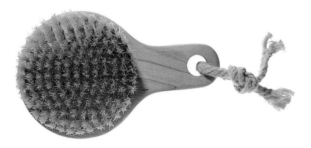

SKIN BRUSHING

On the morning of your juice fast, skin brushing is an excellent way of waking yourself up, stimulating the circulation and lymphatic systems, speeding up the detoxification process, and, incidentally, giving you smooth, glowing skin. It is a very simple procedure in which you sweep a natural bristle brush all over your body before you shower. In other words, you brush dry skin and then wash. The whole process should take around five to ten minutes. Use long, smooth movements, starting at the soles of your feet and gradually moving upwards – always in the direction of your heart. If you aren't used to it, the brush may feel a little rough on your skin at first, but if you use it regularly, you'll soon find it invigorating. There is no need to apply a lot of pressure; the idea is to make the movements sweeping and rhythmic.

How to skin brush: Skin brushing is always done on dry skin, before you shower. Make sure that the bathroom is warm and you have plenty of towels to hand when you get out of the shower.

■ Undress. Sit on a chair or the edge of the bath. Begin with the sole of the right foot. Stroke the sole several times in a firm, rhythmic manner. Continue the movement as seamlessly as possible over the top of the foot, up the ankle and the lower leg, making sure that you cover the whole surface, including shin and calf. Brush upwards, repeating each stroke several times.

■ Stand up and brush the area from the knee to the top of the thigh. Again, cover the area several times with long, rhythmic strokes. Continue over the buttocks to the waist. Now repeat this on the left leg, starting with the left sole. From the top of your buttocks, moving upwards, brush the whole of your back several times up to your shoulders as best you can.

■ Next, brush the right arm. Start with the palm, then back, of the hand, then move from the wrist to the elbow, always upwards. Continue along the upper arm, from the elbow to the shoulder. Repeat on the left.

■ Next, brush the abdomen in a clockwise circle using very light pressure. Continue up to your chest and neck, gently working towards your heart. Your skin should glow. Have a shower and use a body moisturizer afterwards.

AROMATHERAPY BATHS

A bath with the right aromatherapy oils ensures the deepest of slumbers. For maximum benefit, relax in the bath for at least twenty minutes. The water should not be too hot, as this will make the oils evaporate. Afterwards, pat yourself dry gently, so that you do not rub off any remaining oil and leave it on your skin overnight. Some of my favourite oils are:

■ Lavender is safe enough to apply directly on the skin. It is soporific, inducing a deep, tranquil sleep. It relieves headaches and both physical and mental stress.
■ Neroli, extracted from the blossom of the orange tree, is calming and feminine.
■ Rose is expensive but worth it. It induces deep restful sleep, relieves headaches and depression, and rejuvenates!
■ Sandalwood has a warm, woody fragrance. It is an anti-depressant and is soporific. Men often find it more appealing than floral scents.

After the
juice fast

You will be able to continue the effects of the juice fast if you come out of it gently and carefully. After all, there's little point in doing it if you just go straight back to old bad habits afterwards! Even after one day, your digestive system will be more sensitive than usual, so a diet of junk food would do it no good at all.

For one day (or, preferably, two days) after the juice fast, stick to the same regime as for the Preparation Day (pages 104–105). Add a baked potato to your salad meal, if you wish, which you can have with natural yogurt and black pepper and, if you like, a clove of pressed garlic. On the third day after the fast, add some grated cheese to your salad, and have a hearty vegetable soup for your evening meal. After that, build up gradually to your normal – though hopefully, improved – diet. If you are not a vegetarian, add fish to your diet first, and leave meat until last, as red meat is one of the hardest things to digest, and you need to prepare yourself for it gradually.

The one-day fast can be repeated quite regularly, whenever you feel in need of a pick-me-up. It is ideal after a period when you've been overdoing it. Most people find that, far from feeling weak or lacking energy, after a one-day juice fast, they are clear-headed, full of zest and raring to go!

If you feel well after trying this juice fast, you might consider trying out the three-day plan. Like the one-day plan, there are also preparation and follow-up days, but its effects are more profound.

Another way of introducing juice fasting into your life is to have a periodic day off when you drink only juices. If you do this regularly, you will probably need only one day of preparation, and one for returning to a normal diet. You could try this on a once-a-month basis, later increasing your juice days to one per fortnight. One advantage of doing this is that it tends to keep your diet fairly well on track. Because you must prepare for the juice day, and afterwards generally feel healthier and more energetic, it makes you less likely to binge on food that you know is bad for you.

Whatever you decide to do, make sure you incorporate at least one, and preferably two, large glasses of home-made juice into your normal daily routine. This alone will give you a huge nutritional boost and you will definitely see the effects in your looks and health.

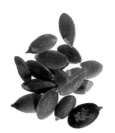
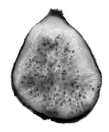
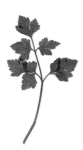
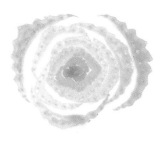

While the one-day plan is an excellent general pick-me-up, the three-day plan is more far-reaching in its effects. It works on a profound level of detoxification and cellular renewal, helping the body to shed old, damaged and diseased cells, replacing them with new, healthy ones. You drink a lot of juice on this fast and, except for the odd moments of craving, you generally shouldn't feel hungry. There is no likelihood of your fading away!

Most of our modern-day diseases are associated with overeating or consuming a diet of overprocessed, undernourishing food. On the three-day plan, the juices themselves provide you with an abundance of concentrated

The three-day plan

vitamins and minerals. Some people may be concerned about the lack of protein in this diet, but your body contains more reserves than you could possibly need. However, the three-day plan is not something that you should undertake lightly. Anyone with a serious illness or eating disorder, diabetes or heart problems should not undertake the fast, and nor should children or pregnant women. Even if you think you are fit, check with your doctor first about your general state of health.

If you feel hungry, this will happen in the first and second days. By day three, your digestive system should be enjoying its holiday and your skin, hair and eyes will be younger-looking. You will also lose up to two kilogrammes (four pounds) in weight.

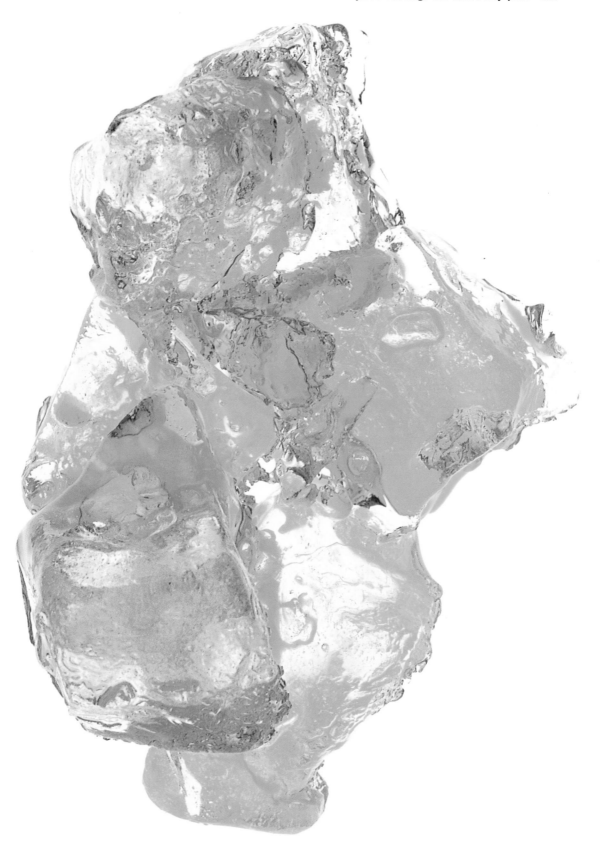

Preparation for the
three-day plan

For the three-day juice plan, you do need to ease yourself into it gently and to prepare for it by having two or three days when you eat only raw fruit and vegetables, with a little wholemeal bread and yogurt. This will give your digestive system time to adjust and begin the detoxification process before the juice fast itself. If you were to start it without preparation, you could suffer some quite unpleasant side effects, as the toxins you have consumed or absorbed over the months and years (from junk food to cigarettes to exhaust fumes to agricultural pesticides) release themselves back into your system before they are finally expelled.

Apart from that, it is quite possible that you may experience some side effects over the course of the three days; however, these are, in themselves, nothing to worry about. They just mean that the detoxification process is working and giving your body the chance to unload the toxins it has built up and not had time to process.

Unfortunately, most of us overload our bodies to such a degree that vital organs of elimination – particularly the liver, kidneys and colon – cannot cope. So toxins are stored, while our bodies concentrate on fighting off infection, or trying to overcome stress or exhaustion. A juice fast gives these organs time to drop toxins and to renew themselves so that they begin to function more efficiently.

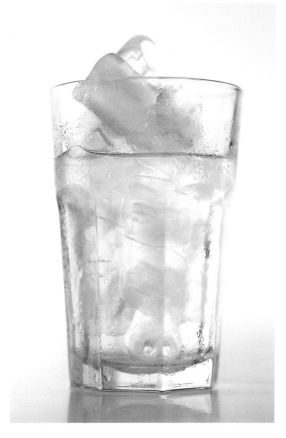

Drinking plenty of water is good for you, especially on fasting days, as it aids the detoxification process.

SIDE EFFECTS

The theory is that toxins hurt twice – once on the way in, and again on the way out. This doesn't mean that you must experience uncomfortable side effects – lots of people have none at all – but that, if you do, you shouldn't worry about them. The most common ones include:

Furry tongue	■ Everyone gets this, almost as soon as they miss the first meal, but it's just a sign that the detoxification is working. Clean your teeth regularly and, if you like, buy a tongue scraper from your health shop (a spoon is also useful for scraping the tongue) and use it – gently – two or three times a day.
Spots (pimples)	■ This is my own most frequent reaction, and just shows that toxins are being eliminated through the skin. This is why you should have one or two baths or showers daily and it is, in any case, a brief problem.
Headache	■ This is another common reaction, particularly if you are prone to headaches or migraines generally. Try not to take painkillers, and drink extra water and rest instead. Massaging lavender oil into the temples and scalp also helps.
Feeling Cold	■ Another thing that happens to everyone is that you feel cold, which is inevitable when you consider that you are not taking in any solid food to act as fuel to keep you warm. It can be a blessing if the weather is hot. If not, wrap up and keep your surroundings well heated.
Tiredness	■ You may feel tired – in which case, rest whenever you need to – although you are just as likely to feel boundless energy.
Flu and cold	■ You may have a runny nose or odd aches and pains, but they are not usually a sign that you are actually suffering from an infection; they merely signal detoxification. Again, rest, drink plenty of water and they should pass quickly.
	All of these side effects are symptoms that your body is detoxifying and, for the vast majority of people, they pass quickly. One way to speed up the process is to assist it by drinking extra water, taking gentle exercise and trying some of the other eliminative treatments, which are worth doing anyway, since they are a pleasure in themselves.

The three days
before the fast

The three-day plan is a deeply cleansing and rejuvenating process that will act as a complete detoxification and beauty treatment. Afterwards, your skin will take on a special bloom, while you should also experience a burst of energy and be a few pounds lighter! However, such magic cannot be worked in the core three days alone, and it is important that you build up to them carefully for two to three days, and to give yourself the same amount of time after the fast to get back to normal at the end of the course.

Throughout this fast, there are some things that must be avoided altogether if the detoxification is to work. These are:

Tea and coffee: These contain caffeine, which inhibits the proper assimilation of the juice nutrients. It also encourages a build-up of one of the least desirable heavy metals, cadmium, within the system. As a stimulant, it should be avoided, in any case, during a juice fast. There are also indications that it is linked with raised blood pressure. Finally, it is a very effective diuretic which robs you of fluids and precious minerals like magnesium that pass out of the body in the urine. Most cola drinks contain caffeine, too, as well as sugar and other undesirable additives.

Alcohol: This should be avoided on two counts: first, it dehydrates the body, which interferes with its ability to detoxify. Second, it

prevents the liver – probably the body's single most important organ of detoxification – from ridding itself of stored toxins by giving it new ones to deal with.

Cigarettes: This is so obvious, it doesn't really need to be said, since cigarettes are one of the most toxic substances your body is likely to encounter on a regular basis. Avoid passive smoking by ensuring that your environment is cigarette free. If you are currently a smoker, you may find this plan a good way to overcome your nicotine addiction.

Drugs: If you are taking long-term prescribed drugs, it is essential that you check with your doctor before you stop using them. However, over-the-counter drugs (painkillers for headaches, for instance) should be avoided, as should recreational drugs.

Everything you need is listed in the plan, so stick to it as closely as you can. If you do get tempted and, in a moment of weakness, eat something you shouldn't, don't give up, just try not to do it again. The more closely you keep to the plan, the more successful it will be. The preparation days for the three-day fast are similar to those for the one-day plan and are arranged like this:

PREPARATION DAYS

8am ■ When you wake up, drink a cup of hot water to flush out the kidneys. Before breakfast, skin brush and shower. For breakfast, have a bowl of natural yogurt with pumpkin, sesame and sunflower seeds, sweetened with a teaspoon of honey, if you like, a cup of herbal tea (see page 105) and a glass of carrot and apple juice.

10am ■ A large glass of water and an apple.

12pm ■ This is your main meal. Make a salad as in the one-day plan, with two pieces of wholemeal bread, and two large glasses of water or herbal tea.

2pm ■ Fruit juice – choose one with grape, plum, kiwi, pear, melon or strawberry.

4pm ■ Water or herbal tea – drink as much as you like throughout the afternoon.

6pm ■ Vegetable juice – choose from tomato, spinach, beetroot or avocado.

7pm ■ Fruit supper as for the one-day plan preparation day (see page 104).

9pm ■ Glass of water or herbal tea.

10pm ■ Try to get to bed early, as your body needs to rest so that it can start its night-time detoxification. Have an aromatherapy bath, if it helps you to sleep (see page 108).

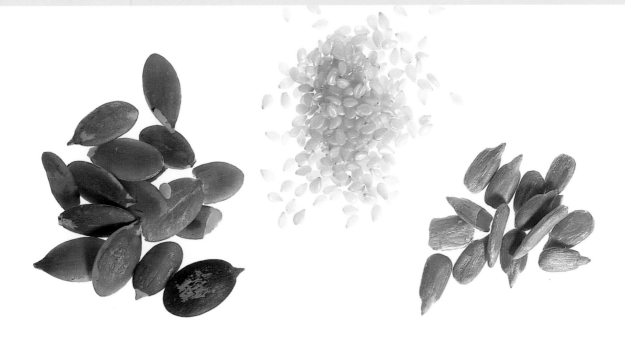

The
juice-only days

It's a good idea to plan juice-only days so that they take place over a long weekend, or a time when you don't have lots of commitments. It's not that they are gruelling; it's just that the more time you can devote to yourself at this time, the more you will get out of the fast. As you will see, there are several other things you can do besides drinking juices, all of which are aimed at making the detoxification process more profound and effective. Opposite is a plan for a three-day juice-only fast.

Except for the early afternoons, the three days follow a very similar pattern. Try to vary the juices each day in order to ingest the widest possible spread of nutrients.

You don't have to carry out the various treatments suggested here, but they will make the fast work even better if you do. Exercising in the morning will help your body to wake up and shed its stored toxins more readily. The relaxation or meditation part of the day is equally important, and helps to reduce stress (which itself can act on the body as a toxin). This is often easily learned while juice-fasting; as the body becomes calmer the mind follows suit.

Finally, remember that one of the most important elements in this plan is getting enough sleep. If you feel tired, have a nap or rest, and try to get to bed early during the juice fast. The more your body rests, the more opportunity it has to repair itself, and the more refreshed and energized you will feel as a result.

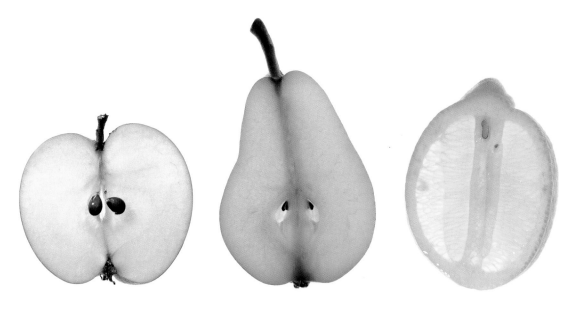

■ DAY ONE

8am	When you wake up, as always, drink a cup of hot water to flush out the kidneys. If you like, you can add the juice of half a lemon to this, which makes it a very cleansing drink. Don't do this, however, if you have very sensitive teeth, as it can damage the enamel.
8.30am	Skin brush and shower, with alternating showers (see pages 108 and 118).
9am	Have a glass of vegetable juice. Choose from carrot, beetroot, broccoli or spinach.
9.30am	This is a good time to do some gentle exercise, such as yoga or stretching. It doesn't have to be too vigorous. Relax for at least ten minutes at the end.
10.30am	A large glass of water or a herb tea.
12pm	A large glass of fruit juice. Choose from pawpaw, pineapple, mango, kiwi or melon.
2pm	Have a walk in the fresh air for half an hour, preferably in a park or in the countryside.
3pm	A large glass of water or a herbal tea.
4pm	A large glass of carrot and apple juice.
5pm	Relaxation or meditation session (see page 118).
7pm	Calming and cleansing vegetable juice using a lettuce-based drink.
8pm	Glass of water or herbal tea.
9pm	Deep-cleansing bath (see pages 118–119).
10pm	Try to get to bed early, as your body needs to rest so that it can start its night-time detoxification.

■ DAY TWO

8am–12pm	As Day One.
2pm	This is a good day to have a treatment that will help with the detoxification and make you feel pampered at the same time. Have a massage (see pages 119–120 for which type).
3–10pm	Repeat, as for Day One.

■ DAY THREE

8am–12pm	Repeat, as for Day One.
2pm	Give yourself a deep-cleansing face and body scrub (see page 120).
3–10pm	Repeat, as for Day One.

Treatments and **therapies**

There are a variety of treatments and therapies that will help to encourage the detoxification process, some of which you can do yourself at home. Others will require you to go to your local health club or alternative therapist, which you will probably need to arrange in advance.

ALTERNATING SHOWERS

Alternating showers are a form of hydrotherapy. They stimulate the circulation of the blood and the lymph, nervous and immune systems, and so promote the body's shedding of toxins. For this reason, it's a good idea to have one every morning of the juice fast. It may sound rather daunting, first thing in the morning, but you stand under the cold water for only a short time and, once you're used to it, it actually becomes pleasantly invigorating! However, please note that if you have a heart problem you should not use the alternating shower therapy.

After you have finished skin brushing, turn on the shower so that the water is very warm. Stand under the shower and let the water pour over you for two to three minutes, making sure that your whole body is covered by it, including your face and head. If you are using soap or shampoo, use it now. Then turn the tap to cool or, if you can stand it, cold, and let it pour over you for 15–30 seconds. Turn the water back to hot for another two to three minutes, then back to cold. Alternate for a maximum of three times, and always finish with cold water.

Immediately afterwards, dry yourself quickly and put on a warm gown, then sit or lie down for at least five minutes, and up to half an hour if you have the time.

This is a good treatment to continue on the days just after the fast, as it will continue to promote the detoxification of your body. Indeed, once you're used to it, you may find that you want to continue it indefinitely as a great way to start the day!

RELAXATION

As the body goes into a period of cleansing and purifying from within, it is not uncommon to find that your mind is following the same track. This makes the juice fast a very good time to try relaxation or meditation techniques. There are, of course, a wide variety of different methods you may use, and you may already have your own favourite ones. If so, use them when suggested, or more frequently, particularly if you have any side effects such as headaches. If you've never tried relaxation or meditation before, a good way to get started is to buy a tape that will guide you through it.

RELAXING BATHS

These are very good at night for relaxing your body before you sleep and for stimulating the detoxification process so that it works throughout the night. You can use the same method every night, or choose different ones according to how you feel. Choose from an aromatherapy (see page 108), Epsom salt or mud bath. None of these baths are suitable for washing with soap or shampoo. If you want to do this, have a shower first and then run your bath.

Epsom salts in warm bath water soothe the body and help the joints and muscles to relax. It is also very good for assisting with the detoxification process, because it encourages perspiration.

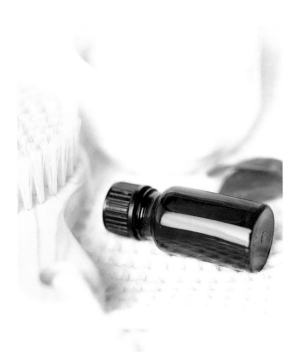

Epsom salts create one of the most cleansing and relaxing baths you can have. It is the magnesium in the Epsom salts which soothes the body and helps the joints and muscles to relax. It is also very warming and makes you sweat out toxins rapidly.

The salts are available at pharmacies and health stores, and come in 2kg (4lb) packs. You simply throw the entire contents into the bath and stir well so that the salts are mixed into the water; check that they are all dissolved before you get in. Lie in the bath for at least 15 minutes and just sweat. You can increase the heating effect by massaging your body with a loofah or bath mitt.

Mud baths contain a high mineral content which has a deeply cleansing effect. One of the most famous and widely available of the therapeutic muds is Neydharting Moor mud (usually known simply as Moor mud). Analysis of the mud has revealed that it is especially rich in decomposed plant life and contains over a thousand plant deposits, including flowering herbs, seeds, leaves, flowers, tubers, fruits, roots and grasses. Approximately three hundred of them have recognized medical properties. Moor mud is both anti-inflammatory and astringent, making it particularly useful for the detoxification process.

Mix the mud well with your bath water, or it will form little globules and not be nearly so effective. Bath water should be warm, not hot, and you should relax in it for at least half an hour. It has a beneficial effect upon parts of the body's skin, so you can also get your face wet with Moor water. The same goes for your hair. Pat yourself dry and go to bed immediately. This is a very relaxing bath, and you usually sleep particularly well after it.

Another well-known therapeutic mud comes from the Dead Sea. This mud is very rich in minerals (principally potassium) which help to regulate the body's water balance. It contains the relaxants bromine, sulphur and iodine. These stimulate cell rejuvenation and repair, while promoting an increase in blood supplied to the skin. In addition, this mud contains small quantities of other minerals (25 in all) which contribute to its general detoxifying effects. Use Dead Sea mud according to packaging directions and relax in the bath for at least 20 minutes. Then rinse with warm water, pat yourself dry with towels and go to bed.

MASSAGE

Massage is a real treat on a juice fast, being both deeply relaxing and a boost to the detoxification process. Don't, however, have an overvigorous massage. Aromatherapy massage is ideal, especially if relaxing oils are used. Another very useful form of massage is manual lymph drainage (MLD), which accelerates the workings of the lymphatic system and reduces the toxins responsible for such conditions as bloating and cellulite.

SALT SCRUB

A salt body scrub clears the pores and sloughs away dead skin cells, so that the appearance and texture of your skin immediately improves. It also stimulates the circulation and the elimination of toxins via the lymphatic system.

For your body, mix rock salt in coarse flakes into a paste with olive or sesame oil. Wet yourself under a warm shower. Take a handful of salt paste and, starting with your feet, massage it into your skin, using your whole hand to make circular movements. Make sure that you scrub the soles of your feet and any hard

areas. Make your way up the legs, using the same circular movements. Pay close attention to the thighs and buttocks; salt scrub is very effective on cellulite. Scrub on those parts of your back that you can, then gently massage the abdomen, then the chest, in a clockwise direction. Finally, scrub your arms and shoulders, and your hands, moving from them to the shoulders (always towards the heart). Step back under the shower and scrub the mixture into the skin as it is washed off.

For your face, mix fine-grained salt into a paste with olive or sesame oil. Wet your face and throat with warm water, then gently massage the paste into your skin. Use two fingers to make small circular movements from the base of your throat to your jaw, starting at the centre and working outwards along the sides. Make the same movements all over your face, avoiding the eyes. Rinse with warm water.

Breaking **the fast**

Returning to your normal routine after the juice fast is just as important as the fast itself. If you overload your body suddenly with too much or the wrong sort of food, you will not only be undoing all of your good work, but you may also find yourself with some pretty unpleasant side effects. So, take it gently and let the detoxification continue for a few more days.

EXERCISE AND TREATMENTS

Continue doing some stretching or yoga exercises and walking in the morning. You may feel like doing something more vigorous, but running or aerobics may be overtaxing; swimming or gentle exercise is preferable.

While on the juice fast itself, heat treatments like saunas and steam baths are not

recommended, but they are excellent for continuing the detoxification process. Steam has a marvellous effect on the skin and will also, over time, help to break down deposits of cellulite. Saunas are good too, especially if you alternate the dry heat of the sauna with cool or cold showers. As with steam baths, saunas relax and promote elimination of toxins through sweating.

However, don't stay in a sauna or steam bath too long – 20 minutes is plenty – and always come out if you feel dizzy or uncomfortable. Lie down and relax as much as possible while you are in the sauna or steam room (but don't fall asleep) and always rest afterwards in order to give the body time to normalize. Don't eat within the hour before or after a sauna or steam bath, and make sure that you drink plenty of water.

■ DAY ONE

8am When you wake up, drink a cup of hot water to flush out the kidneys. Before breakfast, skin brush and shower. For breakfast, have a bowl of natural yogurt with pumpkin, sesame and sunflower seeds, sweetened with a teaspoon of honey (if you wish), a cup of herbal tea (see page 105) and a glass of carrot and apple juice.

10am A large glass of water and an apple.

12pm Make some vegetable soup (enough to store some for the next two days) using any of the following vegetables: potatoes, carrots, onions, celery, cabbage, leeks, turnips, parsnips, sweet potatoes. Two large glasses of water or herbal tea.

2pm Fruit juice – choose from pawpaw, apricot, pineapple, melon, grape or apple.

4pm Water or herbal tea – drink as much as you like through the afternoon.

6pm Vegetable juice – choose from beetroot, carrot, celery, watercress or onion.

7pm Fruit supper, as for one-day plan (see page 107).

9pm Glass of water or herbal tea.

10pm Try to get to bed early, as your body still needs to rest as it continues to detoxify.

■ DAY TWO

Follow the same basic plan as above, but make supper a simple salad dressed with yogurt, lemon juice, and black pepper.

■ DAY THREE

Again, follow the same plan, only add a baked potato, with cheese, if you like, for supper.

■ DAY FOUR AND BEYOND

Return gradually to a normal diet, eating a wide range of fresh, healthy foods, but leaving the foods that are hardest to digest (such as meat) for about a week. By this time, you will be feeling very different – healthier, slimmer, more energetic – and hopefully reluctant to go back to foods that you know will undermine this healthy new you!

Longer **fasts**

Long-term fasting has been used for many years in naturopathic clinics as a means of healing and deep detoxification of the body. The longest juice fast I have ever done was two weeks, but I do one-week fasts regularly. It may be surprising, but, after the first couple of days, I don't feel particularly hungry, and I find the benefits are so great that I like to repeat these fasts up to two or three times a year.

For the main part, however, long-term fasting should be properly supervised in a clinic, such as Tyringham Clinic in Buckinghamshire, England, or one of the many in Germany, Switzerland and Austria, where naturopathy is a particularly well-established branch of health care. It is useful for ailments like eczema, asthma and allergies and is also a very good way of breaking bad habits, such as smoking and other addictions.

LONG-TERM RESULTS

Long-term fasting has remarkable results. The detoxifying and rejuvenating processes have more time to work, and do so on a deeper level, so much so that you can clearly see the changes. Skin tone improves greatly; fasting seems to take years off in terms of fine lines and skin texture, and the eyes become bright and clear, the hair baby soft. Naturally, you also lose weight, although how much depends upon your starting point. Those who are overweight will lose the most (around one pound a day) while those who are closer to their optimum weight will lose less.

Fasting for this length of time also has a profound effect on the mind and emotions, inducing a feeling of calm and confidence. You may physically slow down but, towards the end of the fast, or just as you finish it, you usually feel an upsurge of energy and creativity.

Of course, everyone who fasts has a different experience, and each fast itself is unique. Sometimes a fast can be a real pleasure from start to finish, as if you're on a continuous high. At other times, it is likely to bring out less desirable side effects and may make you feel tired or irritable.

According to naturopaths, this is a sign of a healing crisis. This can take the same form as any of the side effects mentioned on page 113, but as the fast is a more profound one, so the side effects themselves can be more pronounced. They can manifest as flare-ups of any chronic ailment to which you are prone. Eczema, asthma and psoriasis are common examples. The crisis – which usually lasts only about 24 hours – represents a climax of detoxification. According to naturopathy, this is a period of profound healing and, in such cases as eczema or asthma, can often signify the end of the ailment altogether.

WHEN TO FAST

The essential rule for anybody fasting is to make sure that there are no other demands being made upon you. You may feel tired and need to rest and, certainly, you will want to have time and space to yourself in order to gain the most benefit.

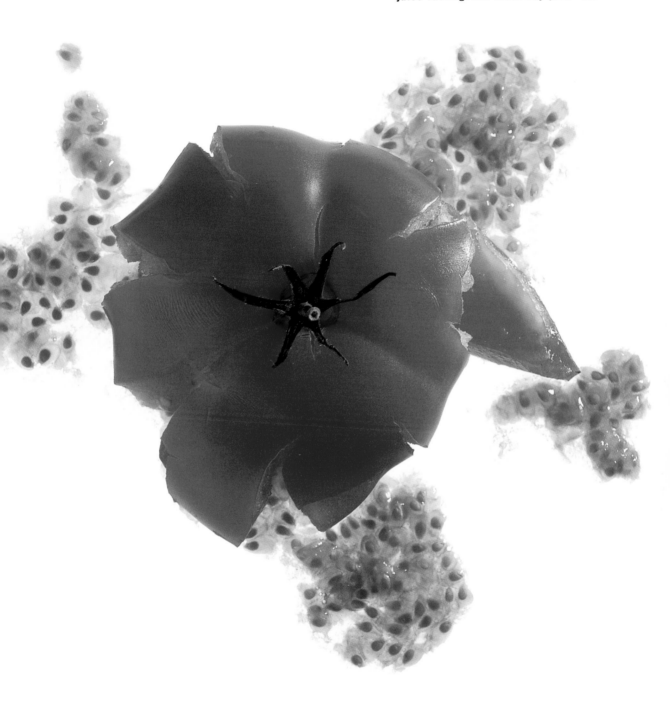

Traditionally, spring is regarded as a good time to fast as the weather warms up and you can get rid of all the effects of cold season comfort eating. You can, however, fast at any time of the year. Do bear in mind that you will feel the cold more, even on a one-day fast. So if you fast in winter, you must make an extra effort to keep warm.

Whenever you fast, and for however long, one thing is certain. You are making a long-term investment in your health by keeping illness and ageing at bay.

Useful **addresses**

UK ORGANIZATIONS:
British Heart Foundation
14 Fitzhardings Street
London W1H 4DH
tel. 020 7935 0185
British Nutrition Foundation
52–54 High Holborn
London WC1V 6RQ
tel. 020 7404 6504
Coronary Prevention Group
Suite 5/4
Plantation House
31/35 Fenchurch Street
London EC3M 3NN
The Institute for Optimum Nutrition
Blades Court
Deodar Road
London SW15 2NU
tel. 020 8877 9993
National Asthma Campaign
300 Upper Street
London N1
tel. 0845 701 0203
National Eczema Society
Tavistock House
Tavistock Square
London WC1H 9SR
tel. 020 7388 4907
Society for the Promotion of Nutritional Therapy
P.O. Box 47
Heathfield
East Sussex
tel. 01825 872 921
The Soil Association
86 Colston Street
Bristol BS1 5BB
tel. 0117 929 0661

Vegetarian Society
Parkdale
Dunham Road
Altrincham
Cheshire WA14 4QG
World Cancer Research Fund
11–12 Buckingham Gate
London SW1E 6LB
tel. 020 7343 4200

US ORGANIZATIONS:
American Association of World Health
1129–2012 st, NW, ste. 400
Washington DC 20036 3403
National Institute of Nutritional Education
1010 s. Jolier St
Aurora, CO 80012
(800) 530-8079

USEFUL WEB SITE ADDRESSES:
Austin Nutritional Research
www.realtime.net/anr/
Center for Nutritional Research
www.bovinecolostrum.com
Food and Nutrition Internet Navigator
www.fnii.ifis.org
International Food Information Service
www.ifis.org
Tufts University Nutrition Navigator
www.navigator.tufts.ed

Further **reading**

**Fresh Vegetable and
Fruit Juices**
Dr Norman Walker
(Norwalk Press, 1999)

The Food Doctor
Vicki Edgson and Ian Marber
(Collins & Brown, 1999)

Skin Secrets
Professor Nicholas Lowe and
Polly Sellar
(Collins & Brown, 1999)

Quantum Healing
Deepak Chopra
(Bantam Press, 1989)

**Juice Fasting and
Detoxification**
Steve Meyerowitz
(Sprout House, 1992)

Ageless Ageing
Leslie Kenton
(Century Hutchinson, 1985)

Fasting to Save Your Life
Herbert N Shelton
(American Natural Hygiene
Society, Inc., 1993)

The Vitamin Alphabet
Dr Christina Scott-Moncrieff
(Collins & Brown, 1999)

Acknowledgements

I would like to offer my thanks to eveyone prepared to be a guinea pig for my recipes, especially my son Christian, an accomplished juicer at the age of seven, and my friends Jane Revell and Diana Craig. I am also very grateful for the support and commitment of Liz Dean and Muna Reyal at Collins & Brown.

Index

ageing 9, 11, 12, 51, 86
alcohol 93, 114
alfalfa 13, 19
allergies 53, 90
anaemia 16, 47, 50, 63, 86
antibiotic effect 61, 78, 80
antioxidants 9, 10, 12–19, 44, 86, 93
apple 14, 30, 36, 46
  mixed juices 62, 63, 64, 66, 70, 72, 73, 74
apricot 12, 14, 36, 50, 53
aromatherapy 95, 107, 108, 118, 119–20
arthritis 19, 56, 65, 77, 87
artichoke, globe 73
asparagus 74
asthma 87, 122
avocado 29, 74

bad breath 87
banana 12, 13, 15, 29, 41, 61
  mixed juices 48, 58, 62
baths and showers 90, 105, 107, 118–19, 120
beansprouts 12, 19, 38, 72
beetroot 13, 16, 67, 85
  mixed juices 68, 72, 74, 80
beta-carotene see vitamin A
bioflavonoids 14, 18
biotin 15, 16, 19
blackberry 14, 60
blackcurrant 12, 13, 14, 49
blood 12, 13, 16, 55, 63, 70
blood pressure 13, 16, 17, 71, 93
blood sugar 44
blueberry 18
bones 11, 12, 13, 17, 72
breastmilk 16, 50

broccoli 12, 13, 16, 68
bromelian 15, 49, 61
Brussels sprouts 19

cabbage 12, 13, 16, 36, 69, 71, 81
caffeine 105, 114
calcium 12, 13, 14–19, 75
camomile tea 105
cancers 9, 12, 44, 86, 87–8, 110
carotene 12, see also vitamin A
carrot 12, 13, 16, 66, 85, 91
  mixed juices 58, 70, 71, 73–77, 80
catarrh 78
cauliflower 12, 19, 81
celeriac 13, 17, 77, 78
celery 12, 13, 16, 70, 71, 77, 79, 89
cellular function 13, 17, 58
cellulite 88
chard 68
chemical residues 30–31, 36
cherry 12, 13, 14, 36, 53, 65
chicory 17, 77
children 30, 39, 40, 44, 52, 85, 91
chives 19
chlorine 13, 15, 17, 19
cholesterol 14, 18, 46, 61, 88
circulation 12, 13, 16, 17, 19, 88, 105
citrus juices 34, 58
cleansing effect 10, 14–19, 90, 104–5
coffee 93, 114
cola drinks 114
coldness 113
colds 19, 64, 80, 89, 113

constipation 16, 63, 89
cooling 89
copper 14, 15, 17, 18
cough 89, 113
cramp 89, 95
cranberry 18, 61
cucumber 13, 17, 67, 76, 78, 79
cumin 41
cystitis 18, 50, 89–90, 105

dandelion 70, 75
depression 11
detoxification 10, 14, 15, 16, 24, 90
  side-effects 113
diarrhoea 90
digestion 10, 12, 14–19, 24, 89, 92–4, 105
diluting 27, 40, 85
diuretics 15, 17, 19
drugs 114

eczema 90, 122
emotions 10–11, 60, 122
energy 12, 13, 14, 15, 16, 44, 85, 91
enzymes 10, 41
exercise 88, 105, 107, 116, 120
eyes 16, 68, 77, 91

farming techniques 30–31
fasting 100–122
  long 122–3
  one day 102–9
  three days 110–21
fennel 17, 68, 79, 92
fever 65, 91–2, 105
fibre 10

fig 18, 63
flatulence 69, 92, 105
flavonoids 14, 15
fluid retention 16, 50, 54, 60, 97
folic acid 12, 14–19, 86
free radicals 9, 86
freezing 39
freshness 28–9, 38–9, 85
fruits 14–15, 18, 44–65

gallstones 88, 92
garlic 12, 13, 17, 44, 80, 88
genetically modified foods 31
ginger 19, 26, 40, 46
  mixed juices 51, 59, 73, 76
  tea 92, 105
ginseng 51
globe artichoke 73
gooseberry 18
grapefruit 18, 58, 78
grapes 12, 13, 14, 36, 52–3, 56
greens 12, 13, 19, 36, 68–9, 81, 89
guava 18

hair 12, 13, 16, 17, 92
headaches 17, 26, 93, 105, 113
heart 9, 12, 13, 17, 86
herbal teas 92, 105
herbs 19, 26, 38, 40–41, 66, 76
honey 40, 41

ice lollies 39
immune system 10, 12, 14–19, 24, 89, 93–4
indigestion 19, 64, 94

iodine 13, 48
iron 12, 13, 14–19, 41, 87

jet-lag 75
juice bars 22
juice days 109
juicers 34–5
juicing methods 32–41

kale 19
kernels 32, 36
kidneys 13, 14–19, 24, 74, 79, 112
  stones 76, 94
kiwi fruit 13, 14, 54, 61, 66

lecithin 41
leek 12, 13, 19, 44, 80
lemon 13, 18, 36
lettuce 13, 16, 36, 72, 73
lime 18
liver 13, 14–18, 24, 44, 112, 114
lymphatic system 16, 120

magnesium 13, 14–19, 89
mandarin 59
manganese 13, 14, 16, 18
mangetout 13
mango 12, 14, 36, 51, 55
massage 95, 119–20
meditation 94, 118
melon 12, 13, 15, 36, 56, 61, 64
menopause 16, 79
menstruation 13, 16, 50, 64, 79, 86, 95
mental health 10–11, 60, 122
metabolism 12, 13
migraine 71, 93

minerals 13, 14–19, 41
mint 19, 66
muscle growth 13

nails 11, 12, 13, 16, 17, 94–5
naturopathy 122
nausea 19, 79, 95
nectarine 15, 53, 59
nervous system 12, 13, 19, 77, 105
nettle 50, 73
niacin *see* vitamin B3
nitrates 30–31
nutrition 9–19, 44
nuts 22, 41

onion 13, 17, 44, 78
orange 12, 15, 36, 46, 58
organic produce 27, 29, 30–31, 36–7

pantothenic acid *see* vitamin B5
papain 14
parsley 12, 13, 19, 76
parsnip 17, 79
passion fruit 12, 13, 18
pawpaw (papaya) 12, 13, 14, 29, 36, 51
peach 12, 15, 30, 36, 57
pear 14, 36, 48, 55
pectin 14
peppermint tea 92, 105
peppers 12, 13, 16, 68, 71, 73
persimmon 57
pesticides 9, 30–31, 36
phosphorus 12, 13, 14–19
pineapple 12, 15, 62
  mixed juices 48, 50, 51, 53, 59, 63
pips 36

pits 32, 36
plum 15, 36, 53, 56, 63
pollution 9, 30–31
potassium 13, 14–19, 75, 89
potato 12, 19, 79
premenstrual syndrome (PMS) 50, 95, 97
pumpkin 12
pyridoxene *see* vitamin B6

quince 64, 69

radish 13, 17, 81
raspberry 13, 15, 64
raw state 10
redcurrant 49, 65
relaxation 87, 94, 106, 118
respiratory system 12, 17, 89, 96, 105
rheumatism 17, 46, 87
riboflavin *see* vitamin B2
ripeness 28–9
rocket 70, 75

salt body scrub 120
salt (sodium) 13, 14, 16, 88, 89, 93
saunas 105, 120
schizophrenia 11
seaweed 12, 13, 19
seeds 36, 41
selenium 9, 10, 13, 86
senility 11
sesame seeds 41
shallots 44
side effects 24, 113, 122
silicon 17, 19, 72
skin 11, 12, 14, 17, 19, 96
  ailments 16, 86, 90–91, 113, 122

brushing 88, 107, 108, 118
skins, washing/peeling 27, 30, 36–7
sleep 72, 94, 105, 116
smoking 12, 87, 88, 93, 114
smoothies 22, 41, 85
sodium (salt) 13, 14, 16, 88, 89, 93
sore throat 19, 71, 96
spices 19, 40–41
spinach 12, 13, 17, 67, 73, 74
spirulina 22, 41, 66
sprouting 19, 38
stones 32, 36
storing 38–9
strawberry 12, 15, 56, 65
stress 9, 12, 44, 90, 93, 94, 96–7
sulphur 13, 16, 17, 18, 19
sunlight 12
swede 17
sweet potato 12, 13, 17, 69, 80
sweetness 24, 40, 41, 44, 62, 85

tangerine 18
tea 93, 114
  herbal 92, 105
teeth 12, 13, 17
thiamine, see vitamin B1
thyroid hormone 13, 48
tiredness 44, 75, 90–91, 113, 116
tomato 12, 13, 16, 69, 70, 72
turnip 13, 17, 75

ulcers 16, 79, 80, 97

vegetables 16–17, 20, 44, 66–81

vitamins 9, 10, 12, 14–19
  A (beta-carotene) 9, 10, 12, 14–19, 41, 77, 86
  B 10, 14–19
  B1 (thiamine) 11, 12, 14, 15, 19
  B2 (riboflavin) 12, 14, 19
  B3 (niacin) 12, 14–19
  B5 (pantothenic acid) 12, 14, 15
  B6 (pyridoxene) 12, 14–17
  B12 12, 19
  C 9, 10, 12, 14–19, 31, 79, 86
  D 12
  E 10, 12, 14–19, 86
  K 12
  see also biotin; folic acid

water intake 13, 104, 105, 107, 117
watercress 12, 13, 16, 40, 70, 71, 77
watermelon 12, 15, 36, 47, 60, 65
weight loss 68, 79, 97, 122
wheatgerm 41

yogurt 41, 85

zinc 10, 11, 13, 14–19, 31